ELDERLY PATIENTS
AND THEIR DOCTORS

Marie R. Haug, Ph.D., received her doctorate in Sociology from Case Western Reserve University, and has been teaching there since 1968. A Professor of Sociology, she is also the director of the University's Center on Aging and Health. Her research interests include studies in doctor-patient relationships, health services utilization by the elderly, and cross-cultural issues in menopause. She has published widely, in books and professional journals such as *The Journal of Gerontology*, The *Journal of Health and Social Behavior*, and *Medical Care*. Her most recent book, *Work and Technology*, was edited with Jacques Dofny of the University of Montreal. Dr. Haug has served on National Institute of Mental Health scientific review panels and in elected positions in regional, national and international sociology professional associations, among them the North Central Sociological Association, the American Sociological Association, and the International Sociological Association.

ËLDERLY PATIENTS AND THEIR DOCTORS

MARIE R. HAUG, Ph.D.
Editor

with the assistance of
M. Powell Lawton, Ph.D.

Foreword by
Robert N. Butler, M.D.

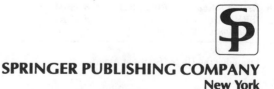

SPRINGER PUBLISHING COMPANY
New York

Springer Publishing Company, Inc.
200 Park Avenue South
New York, New York 10003

81 82 83 84 85 86 / 10 9 8 7 6 5 4 3 2 1

Library of Congress Cataloging in Publication Data

Main entry under title:

Elderly patients and their doctors.

   Bibliography: p.
   Includes index.
   1. Aged—Medical care. 2. Physician and patient.
3. Geriatrics—Psychological aspects. I. Haug, Marie.
II. Lawton, M. Powell (Mortimer Powell).
[DNLM: 1. Physician-patient relations. 2. Geriatrics.
WT 100 E37]
RA 564.8.E43   618.97′023   81-8804
ISBN 0-8261-3570-6   AACR2
ISBN 0-8261-3571-4 (pbk.)

Printed in the United States of America

Contents

Foreword

Recently, a vibrant 93-year-old woman called to express her appreciation over the fact that the National Institute on Aging had adopted geriatric medicine as a major priority. She had lived long enough, she said, to see the development of pediatrics, based, at least in part, on the recognition of the wondrous individuality of children. Now, she felt that medicine would soon discover the equally wondrous diversity of older persons. Hastening that recognition is *Elderly Patients and Their Doctors*. It is a book that reflects the increasing realization by older people, their familiies, and their doctors of the need to examine the doctor/patient relationship.

There is also an increasing awareness of a compelling need to foster the discovery and application of new knowledge concerning (1) health promotion and disease prevention in older persons, (2) diagnostic evaluation of older persons, and (3) care and treatment of older persons. Considering the large growth of the population involved, strikingly little is known about age-related illnesses—their causes, physical and psychosocial consequences, and effective therapies. Also, considering the fact that health costs are escalating at a staggering rate, we must promote the growth of the important field of geriatrics in schools of medicine, nursing, social work and allied disciplines. The complexities of disease and old age have not been appreciated yet in full measure by medical and other health schools. Indeed, this failure reflects a devalued view of older persons, one that is often held in the health professions and manifested by such epithets as "crock," "gomer," "gork," and even "dirt ball." Ageism is part of our culture. Despite its humanitarian and scientific roots, medicine has not shaken itself loose from widespread cultural negativism.

The National Ambulatory Medical Care Survey of 1975 (National Center for Health Statistics, 1978) shows that a family or general practioner spends an average of only 12.6 minutes with a patient of any age. The doctor/patient relationship must be improved. It is built on a minimal time expenditure. Data gathered for "A National Study of Medical and Surgical Specialties" (Mendenhall et al., 1978) show that the duration of encounters between doctors and patients declines with age. Thus, the commonplace statement of doctors that "older people take so much time" is a misperception or a lie. There are also financial barriers when out-of-pocket costs are too high for the poorer patient. Finally, significant numbers of older people do not have their own doctor, partly because people usually choose doctors older than themselves and the doctors then retire and die.

Medical practitioners must recognize the distinction between younger and older patients when making a diagnosis. With the younger, it is relatively straightforward. There is usually one diagnosis. Medical diagnosis becomes exceedingly complex in old age because of multiple pathology, multiple use of medications, and complicating psychosocial factors. The impact of one disease upon another can disguise presentation. The features associated with the aging host may also alter the course of the disease(s). It is more difficult intellectually, but also more challenging.

When I went to medical school in the early 1950s, students met older people mainly on the chronic disease service during course work on physical diagnosis. Older persons were presented—not as human beings—but as living museums. The student became acquainted with auditory evidences of stenotic valves and emphysematous rales. The students rarely saw the patient as a whole person! They were not taught the special sensitivities required in interviewing and evaluating older persons. For example, seldom mentioned were the possibilities that they might have hearing impairments, or fear of being told that they have a serious illness. Variation in, and unusual features of, diseases in older persons were not explained. I did see older patients during my medical school career, but I did not see them in a positive and structured context. Students received no instruction to help offset their avoidance behavior derived from a sense of futility and despair. In retrospect, it is clear today that medical goals of diagnosis, care, and treatment were dominated by the desire for dramatic cure—of discovering the single physical cause against which to direct the unfailing magic bullet. Chronic disease in the aging person did not accommodate this wish.

It is essential that the medical student and the doctor see older people in a variety of settings. Among these should be clinics for health promotion and disease prevention, and facilities equipped for effective diagnosis and treatment of acute and chronic illness—including rehabilitation and individual and family counseling. These should be places where restitution and recovery are goals that are pursued realistically. In other words, medical students should see older people in the context of effective, active and *successful* therapy, with *successful* defined to cover those occasions when palliation is the best that can be expected.

For too many years, many doctors have kept a mystery the special knowledge they possess. This must end. First, the doctor must be a teacher to his patients. The original meaning of "doctor" was "teacher." Second, there must be a new egalitarianism in the doctor/patient relationship—a collaboration in which the natural healing resources of the patient are mobilized to maintain health and combat disease. The aging patient must be an active participant in maintaining the greatest feasible degree of health. This collaborative approach would do much to enhance the relationship of elderly patients and their doctors.

Robert N. Butler, M.D.
Director
National Institute on Aging

Preface

This book on the doctor-patient relationship and the elderly patient is very timely. The public as well as the medical profession is becoming increasingly aware that health care of the elderly involves significant social, political, and medical problems. These problems take their most dramatic form with respect to the very old, who are the most prone to suffer from chronic conditions, to be disabled, and to require long-term care. At least two government agencies, the Administration on Aging and the National Institute on Aging in the Institutes of Health, are currently involved in programs that address the issue of long-term care for the elderly, viewing it within the context of medicine and the physician's role. To those, like myself, who have been intimately involved in long-term care of the aged for a number of years, this heightened interest is certainly welcome. It behooves us, however, to look critically at the medical assumptions that underlie this interest. Accordingly, my views on this book will address its relevance to long-term care.

A significant component of our long-term care system is the patient-doctor relationship. Readily apparent in this relationship is the influential role of the physician, a role strongly rooted in the medical management of acute conditions. Long-term care of chronic conditions, however, amplifies the physician's role, intensifying the patient-doctor relationship.

Many factors account for this situation. For one, the physician often serves as the gatekeeper to the long-term care system because, customarily, the older person's condition is initially viewed by both patient and family as a medical one. Thus, the first professional contact when a chronic problem strikes is with the physician. This contact often takes place in the acute hospital, where the physician's control, as noted by Goss in Chapter 13, is particularly strong. The physician's gatekeeper role is further reinforced by policies of third-party reimbursors who tend to view the chronic, disabling problems of the old simply as medical ones.

The patient-doctor relationship acquires new dimensions when chronic disabling illness strikes. Power is conferred on the physician not only by the "system" but by the patient and family as well. Faced with the often dramatic helplessness of the older person, a lack of knowledge, and a sense of panic, families and patients may abdicate judgment and decision making completely to the physician. While understandable, this may not be in the patient's best interests since judgments and decisions made at this juncture are crucial to the future of the older person.

The demands of the patient-doctor relationship appear to be awesome. Not to be minimized are the constraints on the physician's time and his or her inability to "cure" the chronic condition. This may disappoint and even anger the patient and family, thus creating an unfortunate schism in the helping relationship. As Breslau notes in Chapter 10, the physician may withdraw from the relationship if the patient's own sense of helplessness is projected onto him. The busy physician must be attuned not only to his or her own feelings and behavior but to the patient's anger and depression, which often accompany chronic, disabling illness. Even if physicians recognize these realistic limitations and psychotherapeutic opportunities, they must still contend with the additional responsibilities thrust upon them at this time: to guide the older person to whatever appropriate services and living arrangements exist.

Juxtaposed to the important relationship between physician and patient are an array of long-term care services that are heavily institutional in character. Expensive forms of care, such as acute-care hospitals and nursing homes, are more readily available than community-based services such as home health aides and transportation. An appropriate fit between the system and the individual patient is often difficult to effectuate because of both limited service options and limited levels of care.

This heavy institutional bias both contributes to and is exacerbated by the doctor-patient relationship. Skilled nursing facilities, which make up the great majority of long-term care institutions, have long been viewed as minihospitals. Nursing homes were, in fact, built to avoid the utilization of acute-care hospital beds by chronic patients. The same physician whose influence is enhanced by a gatekeeper role, particularly in the acute-care hospital, often chooses institutional long-term care for the patient as a natural extension of hospital care. The tendency for the physician to view chronically impaired patients within a biomedical disease-oriented framework contributes to a hospital-like solution to the patient's problems. In this regard, it is important to note that there has been little, if any, demand on the part of physicians for an expansion of community-based supportive services.

Two divergent courses are being pursued in an attempt to correct this strong biomedical/institutional bias in long-term care. One course seeks changes in medical practice itself; the other seeks more basic changes in the system of care. The first course is reflected, to some extent, in a number of the chapters in this volume. Engel (Chapter 1) urges that the medical profession and its schools adopt a biopsychosocial systems model of diagnosis and treatment of geriatric conditions as contrasted to the current teaching and practice of the reductionist biomedical approach. He further urges an expansion of the doctor-patient relationship to include the family and significant others, as well as a holistic view of elderly patients and their special attributes as human beings.

Williams, Lawton, and Maddox (Chapters 4, 16, and 6) cite the complexity of the diagnostic and treatment processes and the diversity of the elderly. They note the functional variations and the need of the physician for much more knowledge about the conditions of the elderly, their potential for change, and the variety of settings in which they can receive help to meet their highly individualized needs. In addition, the power of family coalitions, notes Rosow (Chapter 12), needs to be incorporated into the physician's perspective. Coe (Chapter 2) describes the sick role usually adopted by the elderly patient in relation to the physician and the inappropriateness of the role for conditions that cannot be cured. He notes, further, the need for a more egalitarian relationship in which small incremental changes are to be encouraged.

The rationale for these proposed reforms in medical practice is compelling. The physician's role, particularly at the entry point into the long-term care system of help for older persons, is a crucial one. If careful psychosocial and functional assessment as well as an accurate medical diagnosis is undertaken at this juncture, appropriate planning can take place commensurate with the functional abilities and disabilities of the older person and the capabilities of family. If diagnosis and assessment are hasty or incorrect, plans for provision of services may be unjustified, insufficient to help the older persons maintain themselves, and, ultimately, destructive.

There are others who would shift the focus from changes in medical practice per se to more basic systemic changes. While a psychosocial, functional, and holistic model of medical care is highly desirable, its realization within the foreseeable future is unlikely in this country, where medical education would have to be significantly altered.

Instead, it is suggested that a dilution rather than an intensification of the doctor-patient relationship be pursued in the development of long-term care for the elderly. The interdisciplinary team should substitute for aspects of the doctor-patient relationship along the entire continuum of long-term care from the initial stages of a chronic problem through institutionalization if required (see Estes, Chapter 11). Assessment of psychological, social, and functional problems must be made by those practitioners most skilled in these areas. Planning on the basis of this assessment and the medical diagnosis needs to be based on the pooled knowledge of all professionals involved, as well as the desires of patient and family. The most important professional person to the patient and family in ongoing long-term care may be a case manager, who coordinates and monitors a cluster of services. Or it may be a social worker, psychologist, psychiatrist, or nurse counselor who provides ongoing needed emotional support.

The success of a multidisciplinary approach in long-term care has been documented. Given a greater abundance of services, community-based case management systems that seek social as well as medical/institutional solutions to the chronic disabling problems of older people can result in less costly and more satisfying long-term solutions for a significant number of older people.

The benefits of this approach (which would require major fiscal and policy changes) are manifold. Not only does it provide older persons and their families with more varied professional relationships to match their diverse needs, but it frees the energies of the physician to concentrate on the urgent task of making accurate medical diagnoses in lieu of the tendency, described by Kart (Chapter 7) to attribute conditions to the aging process itself instead of to possible disease and environmental factors. The attribution of organic conditions to psychosocial causes and vice versa must be guarded against, as noted by Weiss (Chapter 8). More accurate medical diagnoses in geriatric care are long overdue.

Long-term care is composed of social care, rehabilitative care, psychological care, *and* medical care. The future of services to the chronically impaired elderly rests on a multidisciplinary base and, it is to be hoped, will develop within the context of a social/health care system and a variety of professional relationships. These relationships should depend on individual patient need and preference and not on professional status or reimbursement mechanisms. In this way, the patient-doctor relationship may be appropriately utilized for the optimal benefit of the chronically disabled patient.

Barbara Silverstone, D.S.W.
Executive Director
The Benjamin Rose Institute
Cleveland

Contributors

Samuel Bloom, Ph.D.
Professor of Sociology and Community Medicine, Mt. Sinai School of Medicine, City University of New York.

Lawrence Breslau, M.D.
Assistant Clinical Professor, Department of Psychiatry, School of Medicine, Case Western Reserve University.

Rodney M. Coe, Ph.D.
Professor, Department of Community Medicine, School of Medicine, St. Louis University.

George L. Engel, M.D.
Professor of Psychiatry and Medicine, School of Medicine, University of Rochester.

E. Harvey Estes, Jr., M.D.
Chairman, Department of Community and Family Medicine, Duke University Medical Center.

Isaac Fine
Treasurer, American Association for Retired Persons (AARP).

Amasa B. Ford, M.D.
Professor of Epidemiology and Community Health, and Director, Office of Geriatric Medicine, School of Medicine, Case Western Reserve University.

Mary E. W. Goss, Ph.D.
Professor, Cornell University Medical College, and former editor, *Journal of Health and Social Behavior*.

Marie R. Haug, Ph.D.
Professor of Sociology and Director, Center on Aging and Health, Case Western Reserve University.

Cary Kart, Ph.D.
Professor, Department of Sociology, University of Toledo.

M. Powell Lawton, Ph.D.
Director, Behavioral Research, Philadelphia Geriatric Center.

George Maddox, Ph.D.
Director, Center for the Study of Aging and Human Development, and Professor of Sociology and Medical Sociology (Psychiatry), Duke University.

Victor W. Marshall, Ph.D.
Associate Professor, Department of Behavioural Science, Division of Community Health, Faculty of Medicine, University of Toronto.

Irving Rosow, Ph.D.
Professor of Medical Sociology, Langley Porter Institute.

Ethel Shanas, Ph.D.
Professor of Sociology, University of Illinois, Chicago Circle, and Professor of Health Care Services, School of Public Health, University of Illinois Medical Center.

Barbara Silverstone, D.S.W.
Executive Director, Benjamin Rose Institute, Cleveland.

Edward J. Speedling, Ph.D.
Instructor, Sociology and Community Medicine, Mt. Sinai School of Medicine, City University of New York, and Director, Department of Clinical Evaluation, Mt. Sinai Hospital.

Herbert J. Weiss, M.D.
Associate Clinical Professor, School of Medicine, Case Western Reserve University, and Director, Department of Psychiatry, Mt. Sinai Hospital, Cleveland.

T. Franklin Williams, M.D.
Professor of Medicine, University of Rochester, and Medical Director, Monroe Community Hospital, Rochester, New York.

Introduction

On the dust cover of a recent book on geriatric care there is a photograph of a little old lady and a middle-aged man, presumably a doctor. The little old lady is caressing the man's hand, in a posture of adoration and gratitude. Practitioners familiar with the health care of the elderly recognize that this is as much an erroneous stereotype as another possible picture, of a little old lady angrily whacking a doctor over the head with her cane.

In fact, little is known about the nature of the doctor-patient relationship when the patient is elderly, despite the fact that persons 65 and over constitute a large and growing part of the population. In 1979 there were 24.6 million such persons, just over 11 percent of the total. These figures include 9.4 million 75 years old and older (U.S. Bureau of the Census, 1980). Although demographers' forecasts vary depending on assumptions about medical breakthroughs and subsequent death rate changes, the U.S. Census projections are for 30.6 million people aged 65 and over, and 13.5 million 75 and over by the year 2000 (McFarland, 1978). In the 1970s, the elderly group made disproportionate use of health care facilities, filling a third of the hospital beds and accounting for a quarter of health care expenditures (Kart et al., 1978). There is no reason to expect any dramatic reduction in the elderly's share of the health dollar by the end of the century. Indeed, the increase in those over 75, who are most prone to need medical care, forecasts an even larger bite of that dollar by the year 2000.

Thus, on the basis of sheer patient numbers alone, one might expect considerable attention would have been paid to theoretical and conceptual issues involved in doctor-patient interactions. There are, moreover, other reasons for concern. For example, many of those currently very old have few years of formal schooling, a consequence of immigration waves in the 1920s from countries with limited educational opportunities, as well as tendencies in this country for early school leaving to seek employment during the first third of the twentieth century. The median number of school years completed of those 55 and over was 10.9 in the 1970 census. In that same year, persons 30–34, the cohort reaching 60–64 in 2000, had completed an average of 12.7 years of schooling. A fifth of this younger group has completed four years of college, compared to less than 9 percent of the older (U.S. Bureau of the Census, 1972). Such higher educational levels of future elderly can forecast a more knowledgeable cohort, exhibiting a potentially more critical stance toward medical intervention, with implications for styles of interaction with physicians.

The view that the physician-elderly patient relationship has been a neglected topic can be validated by a search of the medical and gerontological literature over the last years. There has been considerable recent emphasis on the health needs of the elderly and on the poor fit between their needs and the health care system (e.g., Auerbach et al., 1977; Brickner et al., 1975). The imperfect knowledge of physicians concerning special health problems encountered in aged patients has been noted, for example with respect to the unique presentation of some diseases (Kelly et al., 1977), surgery follow-up (Handy & Zakaria, 1977), and drug reactions (Anderson, 1977; Pfeiffer, 1980).

Misdiagnosis and erroneous treatment regimen have been attributed to the expectation that the old are apt to die soon anyhow or that their ailments are "just" due to aging. Some attribute these shortcomings to gaps in medical school training (Gruber, 1977), while others note the emotional and status problems felt by physicians treating the elderly (Cohen, 1977).

Variations among aged patients' characteristics and their possible effect on doctor-patient encounters are also largely ignored in the literature. Indeed, ageism, that tendency to hold negative stereotypes of the elderly which pervades our youth-oriented society, may account for this lack, since the medical profession is not immune to it (Elmore, 1968). Missing in the literature are the implications of the distinction between the young-old and the old-old (Neugarten, 1974). Rather, from the emphasis on dying, mental confusion, and fragility, some sources seem to consider that all elderly are either moribund (Lasagna, 1969) or near senility (Woods & Britton, 1977), despite the fact that most old people consider themselves in reasonably good health (Shanas, 1980).

The context of physician-elderly interaction is another relevant issue. For example, multiple problems tend to call for multiple services, often from a team in which the physician is only one member. Thus, the difficulties of interdisciplinary integration of care are overlaid on the problematics of the interaction situation. On the other hand, the elderly patient is apt to bring to the encounter a "team" of his or her own, consisting of family or other members of a support network, adding another complexity to the health care scene.

Still another contextual factor is the location where care is given. Physicians may see older patients in nursing homes, as well as in offices and hospitals, and even occasionally in their own homes. The impact of these varying locales on the relationship has been suggested by Miller et al. (1976), who found negative stereotyping of nursing homes by physicians and disinterest in the care of ill aged in institutions.

The geriatric literature, in short, has paid little attention to issues affecting the doctor-patient relationship or to the nature of the relationship itself. There are a few exceptions, some presenting contradictory views. Thus, Bogdonoff (1970) warns physicians not to show their disappointment when elderly patients fail to respond to regimens. Mead (1977), whose image of the geriatric patient is a person not only ill, but depressed, isolated, and confused, calls for allowing emotional dependence, while Thompson (1965) and Louis Harris (1975) urge that physicians treating older persons concern themselves with maintaining the patient's sense of identity. Perhaps the most balanced view of issues in the interaction comes from a paper by Robert Butler (1978), who points out that the quality of doctor-patient relationships is particularly critical in caring for the elderly because of the likelihood of their presenting multiple and difficult-to-diagnose ailments.

Recognition of the paucity of material on doctor-elderly patient interactions sparked the holding of a symposium on the topic, in October, 1979, under the sponsorship of the Center on Aging and Health at Case Western Reserve University, with support in part by the Cleveland Foundation. The chapters in this volume are edited versions of those presentations. Organization of the book follows a pathway from theoretical conceptualization through to implications of the presentations for practice and for research.

Laying a groundwork for all that follows, George Engel, M.D., and Rodney Coe, Ph.D. outline models for understanding physician-patient encounters, one from the perspective of a physician, and the other from the perspective of a social scientist. Moving from the general to the particular, Ethel Shanas, Ph.D. (a gerontologist), T. Franklin Williams, M.D. (a geriatric physician), and Isaac Fine (an elderly consumer), present their differing perspectives on the barriers to a successful doctor-patient relationship typical of the current health-care scene.

The factors affecting that relationship are then examined in turn, starting with the impact of patient characterstics. George Maddox, Ph.D stresses the variability of the elderly, including the pitfalls in accurate assessment of their problems, while Cary Kart, Ph.D., reviews the diverse ways in which older persons interpret their symptoms, with potentially dangerous consequences in some instances. Closing this section, Herbert Weiss, M.D., a geriatric psychiatrist, presents some case histories that illustrate problems in elderly patient care.

Characteristics of the physician also relate to the nature of the encounter. Victor Marshall, Ph.D., analyzes in depth the variety of ways in which physician variables affect the relationship; and Lawrence Breslau, M.D., a geriatric psychiatrist, addresses the emotional blocks that doctors face when dealing with the elderly.

The context in which care occurs is not neglected. E. Harvey Estes,

M.D., discusses the meaning of team health-care delivery for patient and physician, while Irving Rosow, Ph.D., shows the complex patterns of relationships that can occur when a third party, a family member, joins the scene. Mary Goss, Ph.D., then reviews situational effects on care-giving, whether service occurs in a hospital, doctor's office, or nursing home. Finally, Samuel Bloom, Ph.D., and Edward Speedling, Ph.D., address the larger context, the changing societal forces that encircle the doctor and his or her patient as they work out a modus vivendi.

Although this book was not designed as a specific guide to practice or as a compendium of ideas for research, the chapters clearly are suggestive with regard to both areas of endeavor. Thus, it is appropriate to offer, as a concluding section, some reflections on implications for practice as well as possible directions for future investigations. Amasa Ford, M.D., and M. Powell Lawton, Ph.D., contribute their thinking on these points as a finale.

There have been several signs recently of national recognition of the need to develop links between medicine and gerontology and to train and retrain physicians in geriatrics. Recent initiatives of both the National Institute of Aging and Administration on Aging emphasize the priority that must be accorded physician training in this area, including sensitizing those already in practice to the unique needs and problems of the elderly. The Rand corporation report (Kane et al., 1980) on future medical manpower requirements documents expected shortages of physicians with geriatric expertise, fortifying the position of those who have been pressing for adequate training support.

As geriatric medicine comes of age, and the numbers of trained practitioners begin to match the needs of the growing numbers of educated elderly, surely greater attention will be paid to the special hazards and opportunities inherent in the interchange between care givers and their older patients. This book is designed as a pioneering effort, a first modest step in charting the issues involved and the problems to be solved.

Marie R. Haug, Ph.D.
Director
Center on Aging and Health

PART I

THE
THEORETICAL
CONTEXT

A physician and a medical sociologist present their perspectives on the conceptual model underlying relationships between doctors and patients as a prologue to a more specific consideration of the variations that may occur when the patient is elderly. Each utilizes a systems approach to the issue, bringing the patient *as human being* into the picture. Beyond those commonalities there are many points of difference.

Dr. Engel criticizes the biomedical model, which claims to be based on science, because it makes no provision for consideration of the person as a whole, nor for psychological or social factors, except when these factors are reduced to physical or chemical terms. His biopsychosocial model incorporates the human being as the center of a 15-level systems hierarchy that extends from subatomic particles at the core through cells, to person and community, and finally to the biosphere as the highest order of system. In order to grasp the situation as a whole, systems-oriented scientists, among whom the physician should be included, will attend to the linkages and interrelationships between person/patient and the other system components in which he or she is embedded. Such an approach avoids the reductionist error of assuming a mind-body duality, an error Engel considers at the root of contemporary views that maintain the incompatibility of science and humanism. Application of the two models to the treatment history of a 55-year-old male who suffers a second heart attack illustrates the risks of utilizing the biomedical model and ignoring the factors surrounding an illness. Engel contends that the whole person approach provided by the systems analysis of the biopsychosocial model is the only scientific model, and that the old biomedical framework has now become a folk model, a dogma.

Rodney Coe focuses on the Parsonian concept of the sick role, one of the set of patterned behaviors making up the total social system. Parsons, however, viewed the sick role as a case of deviance, albeit a form of deviance which, unlike criminal behavior, was not the fault of the individual. In the earlier formulations, the responsibility of the medical practitioner, as an agent of social control, was to end the deviance, that is, cure the illness and thus restore the patient to his or her normal roles in the society. Patients were temporarily excused from these roles as long as they sought and followed professional advice in ending their deviance. Later, in response to criticism that these formulations failed to take incurable or chronic ailments into account, Parsons conceded that the physician's obligation was at least to manage an illness, rather than necessarily to cure it, while the patient's obligation was to defer to the physician's superior expertise and make every effort to adapt to the exigencies of the disease in order to take on former roles to the maximum extent possible.

The reader will note that both this classic sociological concept and the biopsychosocial model thus make a basic assumption: that the physician should be in charge of the relationship with the patient. While Engel argues persuasively for bringing the psychosocial characteristics of the patient and the social environment into diagnosis and treatment planning, the physician remains as the manager and planner. Coe, on the other hand, discusses some recent research and writing, particularly work based on conflict theory, which takes into account patient rights in the face of the power and status differences between the practitioner and the ill individual. These developments at least implicitly question the assumption that the physician should be in charge of the interaction. Coe also gives more specific attention to the implication of these issues for the elderly, noting the possible impact of status, education, and cultural and value system characteristics of older cohorts on their relationships with physicians.

Finally, Coe, arguing that even Engel's biopsychosocial approach is reductionist, merely extending the basis for a pathogenic model, suggests that a new model should be explored, particularly for its relevance to old people. This model, put forward by Antonovsky (1979), is "salutogenic," involving asking not how persons become ill, but how they manage to maintain health, and viewing physicians as only one in an array of health maintaining resources.

What emerges from these two papers on the doctor-patient relationship is the fact that this type of interaction has many interrelated facets. Both medical and social science can contribute to understanding these facets in all their richness and complexity. This book, in later chapters, attempts to make precisely that contribution, with respect to the aged patient. In fact, most of the chapters at least implicitly assume the multicausal systems model. It is a challenge for the development of theory to maintain the richness of such a viewpoint while resisting the temptation to become so global as to make operationalization of variables and hypothesis testing impossible.

1

The Clinical Application of the Biopsychosocial Model*

GEORGE L. ENGEL, M.D.

How physicians approach patients and the problems they present is very much influenced by the conceptual models of relationships to which their knowledge and experience are organized. Commonly, however, physicians are largely unaware of the power such models exert on their thinking and behavior. This is because the dominant models are not necessarily made explicit. Rather, they become that part of the fabric of education that is taken for granted, the cultural background against which they learn to become physicians. Their teachers, their mentors, the texts the use, the practices they are encouraged to follow, and even the medical institutions and administrative organizations in which they work, all reflect the prevailing conceptual models of the era.

The dominant model in medicine, and I refer mainly to medicine and physicians, although the content will be generally applicable, is called the *biomedical* model. The biomedical model represents the application to medicine of the classical factor analytic approach that has characterized Western science for many centuries. The limitations of that model have been considered elsewhere and an alternative model, the biopsychosocial model, presented (Engel, 1960, 1977b, 1978b). The new model is based on a systems approach, a development in biology hardly more than 50 years old, the origin and elaboration of which may be credited chiefly to the biologists Paul Weiss and Ludwig von Bertalanffy.

In this chapter, I will consider how the biopsychosocial model enables the physician to extend application of the scientific method to aspects of everyday practice and patient care heretofore not deemed accessible to a scientific approach. As a result, the goal of the Flexner reform to educate a truly scientific physician will come closer to reality (Flexner, 1910; Engel,

*Another version of this paper appeared in the *American Journal of Psychiatry* 137:5 (May, 1980):535-544, copyright by the American Psychiatric Association. Permission has been received from the American Psychiatric Association for the publication of this version.

1978a). This view expands our horizons in the application of science generally to care of patients rather than any shift in the basic sense from the scientific method of our era. It is more a thorough and general application of the scientific method than a rejection of it.

The most obvious fact of medicine is that it is a human discipline, one involving role- and task-defined activities of two or more people. Such roles and tasks are defined in a complementary fashion. Roles are based on the linking of the need of one party, the patient, with an expected set of responses (services) from the other party, the physician. Broadly speaking, the need of the patient is to be relieved of "distress" rightly or wrongly attributed to "illness," however conceptualized. The expectation of the patient is that the other party, the physician, has the professional competence and motivation to provide relief. In practical terms, the doctor's tasks are: first, to find out *how* and *what* the patient is or has been feeling and experiencing, then to formulate explanations (hypotheses) for the patient's feeling and experiences, then to engage the patient's participation in further clinical and laboratory studies to test such hypotheses, and finally to elicit the patient's cooperation in activities aimed to alleviate distress and/or to correct underlying derangements that may be contributing to distress or disability. The patient's tasks and responsibilities are complementary with those of the physician. The patient's responsibilities are, if he or she agrees, to respond to and cooperate with the recommendations of the physician.

In a broad sense, this characterization of the complementary roles and tasks of the physician and patient applies to all healing and health-care systems, whether primitive folk medicine or modern scientific medicine. Primitive folk medicine is based largely on authority, tradition, and an appeal to magical formulae; modern scientific medicine relies on scientific knowledge and the scientific method as the best means to achieve the goals of health and well-being. Both the successes and the deficiencies of the current scientific approach, predicated as it is on the biomedical model, are currently the subject of lively controversy. Protagonists of the biomedical model claim that its achievements more than justifty the expectation that in time all major problems will succumb to further refinements in biomedical research. Critics argue that such dependence on "science" in effect is at the expense of the humanity of the patient. This is a fruitless controversy that cannot be resolved because it is predicated, by advocate and critic alike, on a flawed premise: that the biomedical model is an adequate scientific model for medical research and practice (Engel, 1977, 1978b).

The crippling flaw of the model is that it does not include the patient and his or her attributes as a person, a human being. Yet in the everyday work of the physician, the prime object of study is a person. Much of the data necessary for hypothesis development and testing are gathered within the framework of an ongoing human relationship and appear in behavioral and psychological forms, namely, how the patient behaves and what he reports about himself and his life. The biomedical model can make provision neither for the person as a whole nor for data of a psychological or social nature, for the reductionism and mind-body dualism upon which the model is predicated requires that these first be reduced to physicochemical terms before they can have meaning (Engel, 1977b, 1978b). Hence, the very essence of medical practice perforce remains "art" and beyond the reach of "science" (Engel, 1977).

Focusing on what the physician does in contradistinction to what the bench scientist does highlights the appropriateness, indeed the necessity, for a systems approach, as exemplified in the proposed biopsychosocial model. For although the bench scientist can with relative impunity single out and isolate for sequential study components of an organized whole, the physician does so at the risk of neglect of, if not injury to, the object of study, the patient. Proponents of the biomedical model often cite this impossibility to deal with a patient as one would an experimental animal in the laboratory to support their argument that medicine cannot ever be truly scientific. In that view, only what the physician can approach in accordance with the laboratory model warrants being called science. But such a contention assumes that the factor-analytic approach of reductionism alone qualifies as scientific. Systems theory, by providing a conceptual framework within which both organized wholes and component parts can be studied, overcomes this centuries-old limitation and broadens the range of the scientific method to the study of life and living systems, including health and illness.

For the clearest and most authoritative exposition of systems in biology one must turn to the basic writings of Weiss and von Bertalanffy (Weiss, 1959, 1940, 1949, 1967, 1969, 1977; von Bertalanffy, 1952, 1968, 1969). Weiss points out that systems theory is best approached through the common-sense observation that nature is ordered as a hierarchically arranged continuum, with its more complex, larger units being superordinate to the less complex, smaller units. This may be represented schematically by a vertical stacking to emphasize the hierarchy (Figure 1–1) and by a nest of squares to emphasize the continuum (Figure 1–2). Each level in the hierarchy represents an organized dynamic whole, a system of sufficient persistence and identity to justify being named. The name itself reflects its distinctive properties and characteristics. Cell, organ, person, family each indicate a level of complex integrated organization about the existence of which a high degree of consensus holds. Each system implies qualities and relationships distinctive for that level of organization, and each requires criteria for study and explanation unique for that level. In no way can the methods and rules appropriate for the study and understanding of the cell as cell be applied to study of the person as person or the family as family. Similarly, the methods needed to identify and characterize the components of the cell have to be different from those required to establish what makes for the wholeness of the cell.

FIGURE 1–1
Systems Hierarchy (Levels of Organization)

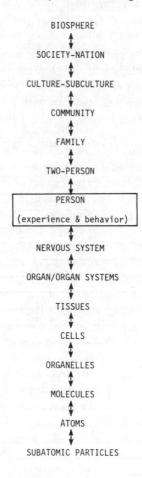

Consideration of the hierarchy as a continuum reveals another obvious fact. *Each system is at the same time a component of higher systems* (Figure 1–2). System *cell* is a component of systems *tissue* and *organ* and *person*. *Person* and *two-person* are components of *family* and *community*. *In the continuity of natural systems every unit is at the very same time both a*

whole and a part. Person (or individual) represents the highest level of the social hierarchy. Each system as a whole has its own unique characteristics and dynamics; as a part, it is a component of a higher-level system. The designation system bespeaks the existence of a stable configuration in time and space, a configuration that is maintained not only by the coordination of component parts in some kind of internal dymanic network but also by the characteristics of the larger system of which it is a component part. Stable configuration also implies the existence of boundaries between organized systems across which material and information flow.

Nothing exists in isolation. Whether a cell or a person, every system is influenced by the configuration of the systems of which each is a part, that is, by the environment. Or more precisely, neither the cell nor the person can be fully characterized as a dynamic system without characterizing the

FIGURE 1–2
Continuum of Natural Systems

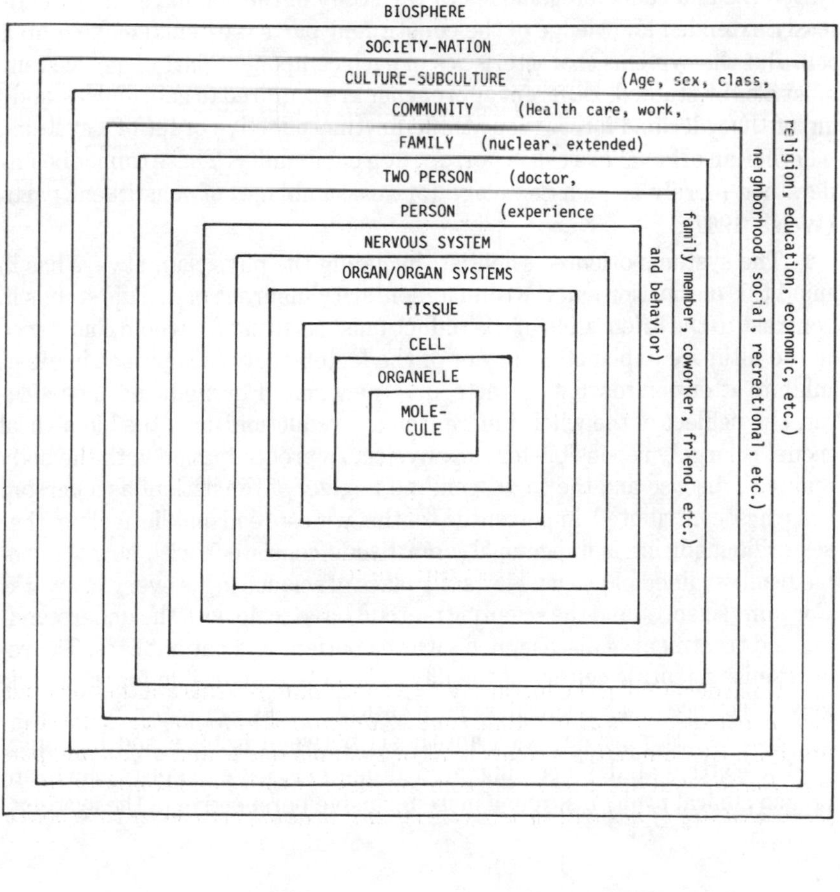

larger system(s) (environment) of which it is part. This is implicit in the labels used. The designation *red blood cell* identifies directly and by inference the larger systems without which the red blood cell has no existence. The term *patient* characterizes an individual in terms of a larger social system. We can think of a patient only in terms of that person's relationships to others representing the larger social systems. Identification of the patient by name, age, sex, marital status, occupation, and residence identifies other systems of which that patient is a component and which in turn are part of the environment.

In scientific work, the investigator generally is obliged to select one system level upon which to concentrate or at least begin his or her efforts. For the physician, that system level is always *person*, a patient. The systems-oriented scientist will be aware that the task is always a dual and complementary one. On the one hand, the constituent components of the system must be identified and characterized in detail and with precision. For this end, the factor-analytic approach has served well. Application of increasingly diverse and refined techniques to the study of the cell have almost endlessly extended knowledge of the constituent parts (systems) making up a cell. But the systems characteristics of each component part of any system must also be studied. Different approaches are required to gain understanding of the rules and forces responsible for the collective order of a system, whether an organelle, a cell, a person, or a community. These cannot be understood merely as an assemblage (or reassamblage) of constituent parts (Weiss, 1967).

The systems-oriented scientist, including the physician, always has in mind this distinction and the complementarity inherent in it. This stands in contrast to the orientation of the reductionist scientist for whom confidence in the ultimate explanatory power of the factor-analytic approach in effect inhibits attention to what characterizes the whole. For medicine in particular, the neglect of the whole inherent in the reductionism of the biomedical model is largely reponsible for the physician's preoccupation with the body and with disease and the corresponding neglect of the patient as a person. This has contributed importantly to the widespread public feeling that scientific medicine is impersonal, an attitude consistent with how the biomedically trained physician views the place of science in his everyday work. For him "science" and the scientific method have to do with the understanding and treatment of disease, not with the patient and patient care. The reductionist scientific culture of the day is largely responsible for the public view of science and humanism as antithetical.

Let us examine how this antithesis between science and humanity might be attenuated, if not eliminated altogether, were the physician to approach clinical problems from a more inclusive perspective of the systems-oriented biopsychosocial model, free of the constraints imposed by the exclusively reductionistic approach of the biomedical model. The hierarchy and continuum of natural systems, as depicted in Figures 1–1 and 1–2, provide a guide to the systems that the physician keeps in mind when undertaking the care of the patient. How this works out in practice may be illustrated by a particular clinical example, the case of Mr. Glover (a pseudonym), a 55-year-old married real estate salesman with two adult sons, who was brought to a hospital emergency department with symptoms similar to what he had experienced six months earlier with a myocardial infarction.

We begin consideration of the model by reminding ourselves that in practice the physician's first source of information is the patient (or some other informed person). Thus, clinical study begins at the person level and takes place within a two-person system: the doctor-patient relationship. The data consist of reported inner experience (e.g., feelings, sensations, thoughts, opinions, memories) and reported and observable behavior. In the instance of Mr. Glover, it was his concerned employer who had recognized that the patient was sicker than he acknowledged himself to be, reported her observations to the doctor, and persuaded the patient to let her take him to the hospital.

How is the clinical approach of the physician influenced by the systems perspective of the biopsychosocial model? With the systems hierarchy as a guide, the physician from the outset considers all information in terms of systems levels and the possible relevance and usefulness of data from each level for the patient's further study and care.

Even such minimal screening data as Mr. Glover's age, gender, place of residence, marital and family status, occupation, and employment already indicate systems characteristics useful for future judgments and decisions. The information that the patient resisted acknowledging illness, especially in the face of a documented heart attack six months earlier, and had to be persuaded to seek medical attention, tells something of this man's psychological style and conflicts. From this alone, the systems-oriented physician is alerted to the possiblity, if not the probability, that the course of the illness and the care of the patient may be importantly influenced by processes at the psychological and interpersonal levels of organization. And of course, the similarity of Mr. Glover's presenting symptoms to those of his recent myocardial infarction prepares the physician to consider systems derangements at the cardiovascular level as well as the symbolic level of "another heart attack."

Such an inclusive approach, with consideration of all the levels of organization that might possibly be important for immediate and long-term care, may be contrasted with the parsimonious approach of the biomedical model. In that mode, the ideal is to find as quickly as possible the simplest explana-

tion, preferably a single-disease diagnosis, and to regard all else as compli-
cation, "overlay," or just plain irrelevant to the doctor's task. For the reductionist physician, diagnosis of "acute myocardial infarction" suffices to characterize Mr. Glover's problem and to define the doctor's job. Indeed, once so
categorized, Mr. Glover is likely to be referred to by the staff as "an MI."

Let us now reconstruct in systems terms the sequence of events com-
prising the acute phase of Mr. Glover's illness. To simplify presentation, we
arbitrarily take as the starting point for this analysis the 90-minute period
during which evolving myocardial ischemia was being experienced by the
patient in the form of symptoms. This and subsequent critical events and
their consequences for intra- and intersystemic harmony are schematized in
Figures 1–3 through 1–9. In each diagram is indicated the system level upon
which the event in question impacts, as well as its reverberations up and
down the systems hierarchy. (Appreciating the unity of the hierarchy, that
each system is at the same time also a component of systems higher in the
hierarchy, highlights the significance of the disruption of the wholeness of
any one system for the intactness of other systems, especially those most
proximate.) These interrelationships are indicated in the diagrams by using
double arrows to connect system levels.

Figure 1–3 depicts the critical events of progressive obstruction to coronary artery blood flow interrupting the oxygen supply and disrupting
the organization of a segment of myocardium. Note that while changes were
taking place at the levels of tissue, cell, molecule, organ, organ system, and
nervous system, illness and patienthood do not become issues until the person level is implicated, that is, not until something untoward is experienced
by the person or some behavior or appearance is exhibited that is interpreted as indicating illness. For Mr. Glover, such changes began around 10:00
A.M. While alone at his desk, he began to experience general unease and
discomfort, and then, during the next minutes, growing "pressure" over
his midanterior chest and an aching sensation down the left arm to the
elbow. The similarity of the symptoms to those of the heart attack six
months earlier immediately came to mind. Thus began the threat of disruption at the person level and with it still another wave of reverberations up and down the systems hierarchy.

Central here is the role played by the central nervous system in the
integration and regulation of the individual's inner experiences and behavior and the physiological adjustments occurring in response to the
processes originating in the oxygen-deprived myocardium. Such cen-
tral-nervous-system-mediated processes are not necessarily in harmony
with one another. Physiological adjustments to myocardial ischemia may
be countered by cardiovascular responses to pain and discomfort as well as

by demand for increased work of the heart resulting from inappropriate behavior.

Mr. Glover well exemplified this incompatibility between psychological and physiological reactions. Whereas the infarcting of the myocardium called for reducing the demand for myocardial work and minimizing such arrhythmogenic factors as excessive catecholamine secretion, the patient's psychological response was to oscillate between alarm and increased sympathetic nervous system activity and denial and inappropriate physical activity (Figure 1–3).

FIGURE 1–3
Event 1: Coronary Occlusion

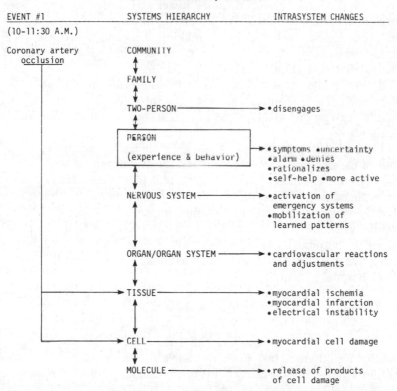

As he was later to report, almost from the start the possibility of a second heart attack came to mind, but he dismissed this in favor of "fatigue," "gas," "muscle strain," and finally "emotional tension." But the negation itself," *not* another heart attack," leaves no doubt that the idea "heart attack" was very much in his mind despite his apparent denial.

Behaviorally, he alternated between sitting quietly to "let it pass," pacing about the office to "work it off," and taking Alka Seltzer. Another employee came into the office, but Mr. Glover avoided him.

When he could no longer deny the probability, if not the certainty, of another heart attack, a different set of concerns emerged as his personal values of responsibility and independence and his fear of losing control over his own destiny gained ascendancy. The new formula became, "If this really is a heart attack (but maybe it will still prove not to be), I must first get my affairs in order so that no one will be left in the lurch." In this way, he tried to sustain his self-image of competence, responsibility, and mastery, but at the cost of imposing an even greater burden on the already overburdened heart and cardiovascular system. In systems terms, feedback was becoming increasingly positive, and a dangerous vicious cycle was in the making. Disruptive processes were gaining ascendancy over regulatory processes, increasing the risk of a lethal arrhythmia (Lown, Verrier, & Rabinowitz, 1977; Engel, 1978c; Mead, 1976). The patient persisted in this determined, almost frenetic behavior for more than an hour until the intervention of his employer brought it to an end and enabled him to accept hospitalization and patient status.

Figure 1–4 diagrams the psychological stabilization that took place as a result of his employer's intervention and the stabilizing consequences for other systems. The intervention, we note, took place within the two-person system, immediately affecting person, and for the moment at least terminated the vicious cycle, thereby lessening impact on the damaged heart of potentially deleterious extracardiac influences. By the time the patient reached the hospital, he was no longer having chest discomfort, he was feeling relatively calm and confident, and was coming to terms with once again being a hospital patient.

How had the employer brought about such a felicitous result? As was later learned from the patient, the employer's approach to Mr. Glover was to commend his diligence and sense of responsibility, even in the face of being so obviously ill, and to reassure him that he had left his work in suitable condition for others to take over. But she also challenged him to consider whether a higher responsibility to his family and his job did not require him to take care of himself and go to the hospital. Intuitively, she had appreciated this man's need to see himself as responsible and in control, and she had sensed his deep fear of being weak and helpless.

By the time Mr. Glover was admitted to the emergency department shortly before noon, he was no longer having any discomfort. But the staff agreed that prompt institution of a coronary care routine was nonetheless justified. This was in fact reassuring to the patient, who had by now accept-

FIGURE 1–4
Event 2: Intervention of Employer

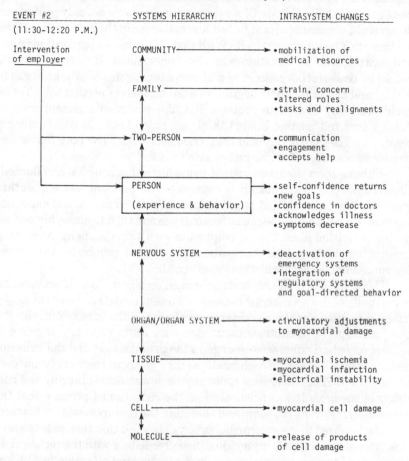

EVENT #2	SYSTEMS HIERARCHY	INTRASYSTEM CHANGES
(11:30-12:20 P.M.)		
Intervention of employer	COMMUNITY	• mobilization of medical resources
	FAMILY	• strain, concern • altered roles • tasks and realignments
	TWO-PERSON	• communication • engagement • accepts help
	PERSON (experience & behavior)	• self-confidence returns • new goals • confidence in doctors • acknowledges illness • symptoms decrease
	NERVOUS SYSTEM	• deactivation of emergency systems • integration of regulatory systems and goal-directed behavior
	ORGAN/ORGAN SYSTEM	• circulatory adjustments to myocardial damage
	TISSUE	• myocardial ischemia • myocardial infarction • electrical instability
	CELL	• myocardial cell damage
	MOLECULE	• release of products of cell damage

ed the reality of a second heart attack. But 30 minutes later, in the midst of the continuing workup, he abruptly lost consciousness. The monitor documented ventricular fibrillation. Defibrillation was successfully carried out, and the patient made an uneventful recovery.

Interviewed a few days later, Mr. Glover was able to reconstruct the events in the emergency department leading up to the cardiac arrest. His account raised doubts that the onset of ventricular fibrillation could be ascribed solely to processes restricted to the injured myocardium alone. Rather, it suggested a major role for extracardiac (neurogenic) influences originating in disturbances at the two-person and person levels. According to Mr. Glover, everything had been proceeding smoothly until the house officers ran into difficulty doing an arterial puncture. They persisted in their fruitless effort for some 10 minutes and then left, explaining only that they were going for help. For Mr.Glover, the procedure was not only painful and disagreeable; more important he felt his confidence in the competence of the medical staff being undermined. With that, his sense of personal mastery and control over his situation was also undermined. Rather than being helped by powerful but concerned and competent professionals, he began to feel himself as victimized by beginners who themselves needed help. Yet he could not bring himself to protest. His tape-recorded comment was: "I didn't wanna tell 'em that I didn't think, ah, that I knew, he wasn't doing it right. . . . They tried here and they tried there. . . . The poor fellow was having such a tough time, he just couldn't get it."

Within a short time, the patient found himself getting hot and flushed. Chest pain recurred and quickly became as severe as it had been earlier that morning. When the staff left to get help, he first felt relieved. But anticipating more of the same, he began to feel outrage and then to blame himself for having permitted himself to be trapped in such a predicament. A growing sense of impotence to do anything about his situation culminated in his passing out as ventricular fibrillation supervened.

This sequence of events is diagrammed on Figure 1–5. It provides an opportunity to draw a contrast between different models and how the model adhered to influence the physician's approach. In the case of Mr. Glover, the judgment to institute without delay an acute coronary regimen is beyond dispute. Differences emerge in the priorities set and the behavior displayed by adherents of each model as they go about their study and care of the patient. The emergency room approach was conventionally and narrowly biomedical. It was predicated on the reductionist premise that the cause of Mr. Glover's problem, and therefore the requirements for his care, could be localized to the myocardial injury. They felt that this, plus the high risk attendant upon such injury, justified proceeding with the technical diagnostic and treatment procedures with only passing attention to how Mr. Glover was feeling and reacting. When the arrest occurred, the staff congratulated each other and the patient on his good fortune. Had his arrival in the hospital been delayed another 30 minutes, he might well have not survived! It was assumed that the onset of ventricular fibrillation at 12:30 P.M. was part of the natural progression of the myocardial injury.

The model used by the emergency staff in their handling of Mr. Glover was based on the factor-analytic design of the controlled laboratory experiment, in which all factors are to be held constant except for the one under study. For the biomedically trained clinician, this constitutes the standard against which the "scientific" quality of clinical work is to be measured. Translated into clinical practices, it is typically reflected in the predilection

FIGURE 1–5
Event 3: Unsuccessful Arterial Puncture

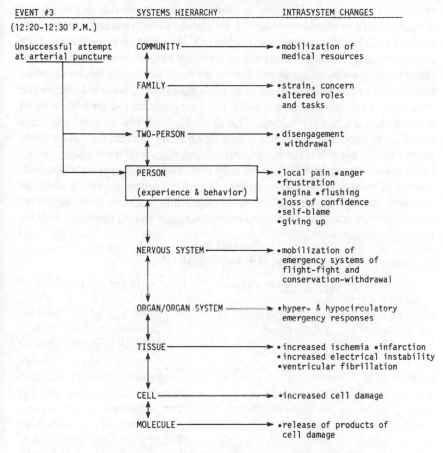

EVENT #3	SYSTEMS HIERARCHY	INTRASYSTEM CHANGES
(12:20-12:30 P.M.)		
Unsuccessful attempt at arterial puncture	COMMUNITY	• mobilization of medical resources
	FAMILY	• strain, concern • altered roles and tasks
	TWO-PERSON	• disengagement • withdrawal
	PERSON (experience & behavior)	• local pain • anger • frustration • angina • flushing • loss of confidence • self-blame • giving up
	NERVOUS SYSTEM	• mobilization of emergency systems of flight-fight and conservation-withdrawal
	ORGAN/ORGAN SYSTEM	• hyper- & hypocirculatory emergency responses
	TISSUE	• increased ischemia • infarction • increased electrical instability • ventricular fibrillation
	CELL	• increased cell damage
	MOLECULE	• release of products of cell damage

to focus on one issue at a time and to pursue a sequential ruling-out technique for both diagnosis and treatment.

A systems approach to Mr. Glover would have differed in notable respects. From the outset, the decision for an implementation of coronary care would have included consideration of factors other than cardiac status, notably those manifest at the person level. The interview of Mr. Glover would have been conducted in such a manner as simultaneously to elicit information needed to characterize him as a person and to evaluate the status of his cardiovascular system. This could have been readily and efficiently accomplished by having the patient report symptoms in a life context, noting acitvities, reactions, feelings, and behavior as symptoms were evolving, as well as his life circumstances at the time of onset. Particularly when considering possible myocardial infarction, the systems-oriented physician is alert to information about person-level factors that might contribute to instability of the cardiovascular system. It would have been valuable as a guide for the physician's personal approach to Mr. Glover's care to learn how the employer had helped him accept the reality of his heart attack and the need for prompt medical attention. And as the coronary care regimen was being implemented, the physician would be closely monitoring the patient's reactions to the procedures, especially in the light of Mr. Glover's documented reluctance to acknowledge a need for help, which would only have been learned through history taking. The difficulty with the arterial puncture would early have been recognized as a risk for the patient, not just a problem for the doctors. Mr. Glover's failure to complain would have been anticipated as consistent with his personality style and not interpreted as acquiescence to what was happening to him. Whether such an approach would in fact have averted the cardiac arrest is impossible to know. But, certainly, sufficient experimental and clinical evidence exists linking psychological im-

FIGURE 1–6
Event 4: Cardiac Arrest

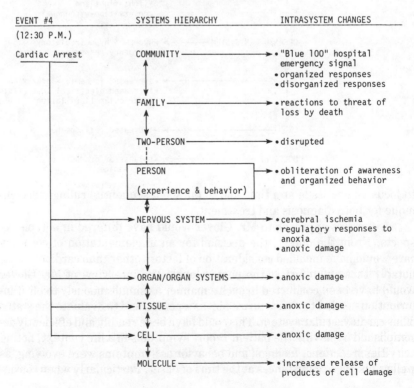

EVENT #4	SYSTEMS HIERARCHY	INTRASYSTEM CHANGES
(12:30 P.M.)		
Cardiac Arrest	COMMUNITY	• "Blue 100" hospital emergency signal • organized responses • disorganized responses
	FAMILY	• reactions to threat of loss by death
	TWO-PERSON	• disrupted
	PERSON (experience & behavior)	• obliteration of awareness and organized behavior
	NERVOUS SYSTEM	• cerebral ischemia • regulatory responses to anoxia • anoxic damage
	ORGAN/ORGAN SYSTEMS	• anoxic damage
	TISSUE	• anoxic damage
	CELL	• anoxic damage
	MOLECULE	• increased release of products of cell damage

passe, as displayed by Mr. Glover, and increased risk of lethal arrhythmias, especially with preexisting myocardial electrical instability (Engel, 1971; Lown, Verrier, & Rabinowitz, 1977).

Further elaboration of the biopsychosocial model as applied to the care of Mr. Glover may be found in Figures 1–6 through 1–9, which diagram in sequence the cardiac arrest, defibrillation, and eventual stabilization of the in-

FIGURE 1–7
Event 5: Successful Defibrillation

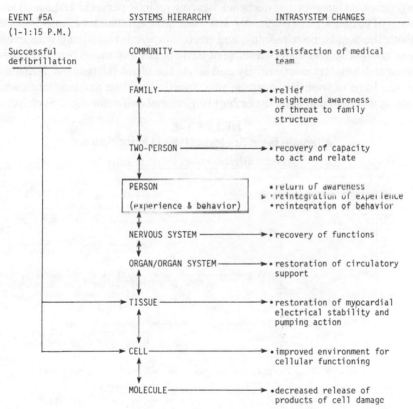

EVENT #5A	SYSTEMS HIERARCHY	INTRASYSTEM CHANGES
(1-1:15 P.M.)		
Successful defibrillation	COMMUNITY	• satisfaction of medical team
	FAMILY	• relief • heightened awareness of threat to family structure
	TWO-PERSON	• recovery of capacity to act and relate
	PERSON (experience & behavior)	• return of awareness • reintegration of experience • reintegration of behavior
	NERVOUS SYSTEM	• recovery of functions
	ORGAN/ORGAN SYSTEM	• restoration of circulatory support
	TISSUE	• restoration of myocardial electrical stability and pumping action
	CELL	• improved environment for cellular functioning
	MOLECULE	• decreased release of products of cell damage

jured myocardium. With the aid of these diagrams, the reader can readily visualize how events or circumstances at system levels above person, whether originating at those levels or occurring in response to person-level illness-related processes, may in turn impinge on the person, and the implications of such for the stability of lower-level systems.

The systems-oriented physician is conscious of responsibilities to the patient and to the family and significant others. At least for the duration of the illness, the two-person system—doctor-patient—is interposed between the patient and the others constituting his social environment. Much business ordinarily conducted directly between the patient and others now filters through the doctor, to whom all parties look for counsel. This is true even when the doctor is not directly consulted, as when people invoke their notion of the doctor's view in his absence, rightly or wrongly. It is especially with respect to these system levels that the contrast between the biomedical and biopsychosocial models is the greatest. For the biomedically trained physician, judgments and decisions bearing on interpersonal and social aspects of patients' lives commonly are made with a minimum of information about the people, relationships, and circumstances involved and with even less knowledge and understanding of basic principles underlying interpersonal and social transactions. By and large, the physician reaches decisions on the basis of tradition, custom, prescribed rules, compassion, intuition, common sense, and sometimes highly personal self-reference. Such pro-

FIGURE 1–8
Alternate Event 5: Unsuccessful Defibrillation

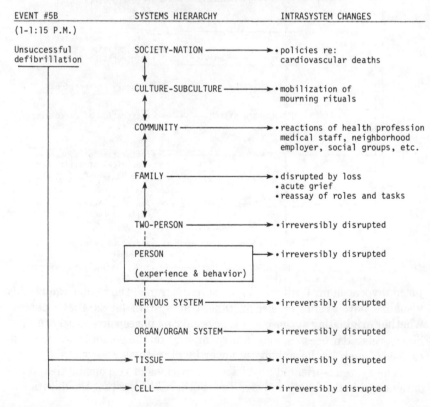

EVENT #5B	SYSTEMS HIERARCHY	INTRASYSTEM CHANGES
(1-1:15 P.M.)		
Unsuccessful defibrillation	SOCIETY-NATION	• policies re: cardiovascular deaths
	CULTURE-SUBCULTURE	• mobilization of mourning rituals
	COMMUNITY	• reactions of health profession medical staff, neighborhood employer, social groups, etc.
	FAMILY	• disrupted by loss • acute grief • reassay of roles and tasks
	TWO-PERSON	• irreversibly disrupted
	PERSON (experience & behavior)	• irreversibly disrupted
	NERVOUS SYSTEM	• irreversibly disrupted
	ORGAN/ORGAN SYSTEM	• irreversibly disrupted
	TISSUE	• irreversibly disrupted
	CELL	• irreversibly disrupted

cesses involving the person and supraperson levels, often of crucial importance for the patient and for the significant others, remain outside the realm
of science and critical inquiry. Not so for the biopsychosocially oriented physician, who recognizes that to serve the patient best, higher-level-system
occurrences must be approached with the same rigor and critical scrutiny
that are applied to systems lower in the hierarchy. This means that the physician identifies and evaluates the stabilizing and destabilizing potential of
events and relationships in the patient's social environment, not neglecting

FIGURE 1–9
Event 6: Myocardial Stabilization

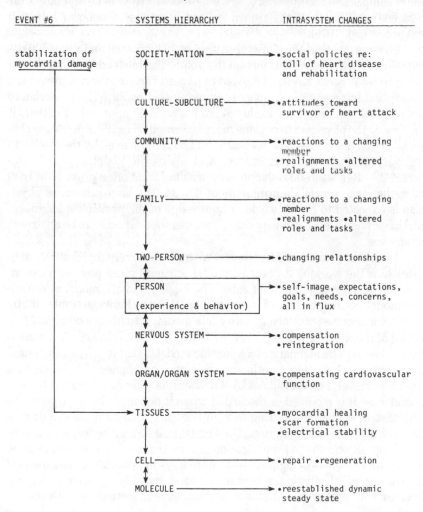

EVENT #6	SYSTEMS HIERARCHY	INTRASYSTEM CHANGES
stabilization of myocardial damage	SOCIETY-NATION	•social policies re: toll of heart disease and rehabilitation
	CULTURE-SUBCULTURE	•attitudes toward survivor of heart attack
	COMMUNITY	•reactions to a changing member •realignments •altered roles and tasks
	FAMILY	•reactions to a changing member •realignments •altered roles and tasks
	TWO-PERSON	•changing relationships
	PERSON (experience & behavior)	•self-image, expectations, goals, needs, concerns, all in flux
	NERVOUS SYSTEM	•compensation •reintegration
	ORGAN/ORGAN SYSTEM	•compensating cardiovascular function
	TISSUES	•myocardial healing •scar formation •electrical stability
	CELL	•repair •regeneration
	MOLECULE	•reestablished dynamic steady state

how the destabilizing effects of the patient's illness on others may feed back as a further destabilizing influence on the patient. Consider the responsibilities that Mr. Glover's physician would have had to face, for example, had Mrs. Glover herself fallen ill—or even died—under the strain of her husband's illness and almost death. Consider, too, how information about Mrs. Glover, readily available to the physician skilled at observation and conscious of its value, would enable him or her to recognize her vulnerabilities and hence avert breakdown and illness. The continuity of systems makes attention to Mrs. Glover's well-being a necessary element in Mr. Glover's care. For the biopsychosocially oriented physician, this is not merely a matter of compassion and humanity, as some would have us believe, but one for rigorous application of the principles and practices of science, a human science (Mead, 1976).

Some argue that the biopsychosocial model imposes an impossible demand on the physician. This misses the point. The model does not add anything to what is not already involved in patient care. Rather, it provides a conceptual framework and a way of thinking that enables the physician to act rationally in areas now excluded from a rational approach. Further, it motivates the physician to become more informed and skillful in the psychosocial areas, disciplines now seen as alien and remote even by those who intuitively recognize their importance. And finally, the model serves to counteract the often wasteful reductionist pursuit of what often prove to be trivial rather than crucial determinants of illness. The biopsychosocial physician is expected to have a working knowledge of the principles, language, and basic facts of each relevant discipline; he is not expected to be an expert at any one.

I hope the example of Mr. Glover, with all of its oversimplification, indicates how the working conceptual model utilized by the physician can influence the approach to patient care. The biopsychosocial model is a scientific model. So, too, was the biomedical model. But as Fabrega points out, by now it has become transformed into a folk model, actually the dominant folk model of the western world (Fabrega, 1975). As such, it has come to constitute a dogma. The hallmark of a scientific model is that it provides a framework within which the scientific method may be applied. The value of a scientific model is measured not by whether it is right or wrong but by how useful it is. It is modified or discarded when it no longer helps to generate and test new knowledge. Dogmas, in contrast, maintain their influence through authority and tradition. They resist change and, hence, tend to promote opposition and the promulgation of rival dogmas by dissident figures. The counterdogmas being put forth these days in opposition to biomedical dogma are called holistic and humanistic medicine. They qualify as dogmas because they eschew the scientific method, leaning instead on faith and belief systems handed down from remote and obscure or charismatic authority figures. They place science and humanism in opposition. But as the history of the biomedical model itself has shown, progress is made only where the scientific method is applied. The triumphs of the biomedical model all have been in the areas for which the model has provided a suitable framework for scientific study. The biopsychosocial model extends that framework to heretofore neglected areas.

2
The Sick Role Revisited

RODNEY M. COE, Ph.D.

The task of this chapter, as indicated by the title, is to revisit the concept of the sick role. Although there were some important antecedents, the conceptualization that is the point of reference here is that of Talcott Parsons (1951). This chapter will review briefly the principal elements of the concept and trace in more detail some developments in theory and research that the concept has stimulated. Finally, some implications of the revisited sick role for doctors and elderly patients will be noted.

Antecedents of the Sick Role

It may be useful to remember that Parsons' analysis of the sick role was only one illustration, albeit an important one, of his broader conceptualization of society as a social system. This broader theoretical interest was examined initially in *The Structure of Social Action*, which appeared in 1937. Even this early formulation, however, had been influenced by Lawrence Henderson, a physician and older colleague of Parsons at Harvard. Henderson was especially important not only because of his contributions to systems theory as a prize-winning physiologist and his later application of these principles to the analysis of society, but also because his analysis of the doctor-patient relationship as a social system was an immediate precursor to Parsons' analysis (Henderson, 1935).

One further digression may also be of interest. The nature of the doctor-patient relationship has been studied and written about since antiquity. For Western medicine, one obvious starting place is the Hippocratic Oath, which contains rather explicit prescriptions and proscriptions of behavior, at least for the physician. In other places, such as the *Precepts and Aphorisms* written 2,500 years ago, or in writings from other eras such as the Renaissance and succeeding centuries, one finds statements about expected behavior by physicians and patients. Some of the elements of these early descriptions are still important in the concept of the sick role. For example, the first code of ethics of the American Medical Association, published in 1847, had this to say about the duties of physicians:

- behave in a professional manner so as "to inspire the minds of patients with gratitude, respect and *confidence*.
- maintain complete *confidentiality* of information.
- don't abandon *incurable* patients.
- obtain *consultation* in difficult cases.

According to the AMA, the patients also had some duties:

- choose only regular trained and certified *professionals*.
- faithfully and unreservedly *communicate* information about self.
- *obedience* to physician's orders should be prompt and implicit.
- don't shop around for other advice; stay with one physician (Reiser, Dyck, & Curran, 1977).

Many of these dicta appear again in the modern expression of expectations of the sick role for the doctor and patient.

The Concept of the Sick Role

Parsons' initial concept of the sick role is well known; only a brief statement is necessary here. It is important to recall that his interest at the time was on deviant behavior and how mechanisms of social control functioned in social systems. Illness, undifferentiated along its biological and social dimensions, was seen as a special case of deviant behavior defined as nonperformance of normal roles. It was a special case of deviance in that the patient was not at fault for becoming ill. Yet, some institutionalized means were necessary for maintaining control and "correcting" the dysfunctional aspects even of nonnegligent deviance. This was the responsibility of the medical profession, and the physician was viewed as the agent of control. Parsons described the relationship between doctor and patient as inherently unequal in status and power because of the superior knowledge and skills of the doctor. The discrepant status notwithstanding, the patient could not be forced to comply, but had to be motivated to do so. Thus, the functioning of this relationship depended upon what we generally describe as professional behavior on the part of the doctor, confidence or trust in the doctor on the part of the patient, and mutual expectations of satisfactory outcomes of treatment. A critical theoretical element was the assumption of explicit and shared norms governing the behavior of both parties as well as expectations for positive outcomes of the encounter.

For the physician, Parsons described norms of "functional specificity," "collectivity orientation," "affective neutrality," and the like that permitted the patient to assume a dependent status without fear of being exploited by the physician. "Functional specificity" means that the physician should pay attention to those matters related to the problem and not get involved in things that are unrelated to it, such as sex, race, or status. "Collectivity orientation" is another way of calling for putting the patient's best interests first and the doctor's interests second. "Affective neutrality" means the avoidance of emotional involvement. For the patient, dependency brought with it a validation of being sick and a temporary exemption from performing normal role duties. However, the patient was obliged not only to seek competent help but to understand that being ill was an undesirable state and that one should want to recover health as quickly as possible and resume one's normal roles.

In anticipation of later discussion, it should be noted that Parsons modified his conceptualization of the sick role in some of his later writings. These changes occurred partly as his theoretical framework evolved and partly in response to criticisms of the original formulation. For example, the concepts of deviance and social control were thought to be tied too closely to characteristics of acute disorders and not accurately to reflect the nature of the interaction when the presenting problem was a chronic condition (Coe & Wessen, 1965). Parsons' concepts of deviance and control now appear to have given way to concepts of *adaptation* and *management*, which can incorporate characteristics of both acute and chronic illnesses. The moral imperatives that health is good and illness is bad are maintained, but motivation to "get well" is extended to "managing disability." Parsons has stated:

> . . . the health care agent, notably the physician, is conceived as reinforcing his patient's motivation to minimize illness and it disabilities. In the case of acute illness, the meaning of this is relatively simple: it is the physician's obligation to reinforce patient's motivation to recover. In a case of chronic illness, like diabetes, the corresponding obligation is to reinforce the patient's motivation to minimize the curtailment of his capacities because of his pathological condition, even though that condition cannot be eliminated in the sense of total cure. [Parsons, 1975:269]

In another place, Parsons restates his assumption of asymmetry in the doctor-patient relationship, but goes on to say that this does not limit the patient to a passive role. Rather, patients can interact with physicians over resolution of their illness at several levels of activity, limited only by the character of the social organization in which the encounter takes place. Parsons felt that the inherent differences in status are least dysfunctional when the encounter takes place in a setting that is governed by a collegial association, for example when physicians themselves become patients. Stated this way, Parsons rejects alternative models such as the market, bureaucratic, and democratic models that were implicit in criticisms of his earlier work (Parsons, 1976). Thus, Parsons' concept of the sick role as a keystone to understanding the physician-patient relationship has matured since its original statement more than 25 years ago. Let us review some major contributions to the evolution of this concept.

Developments in Theory

One early critique focused on the passive nature of patient behavior implicit in the original concept of the sick role. Szasz and Hollender (1956) argued that a passive patient role was only one type of model and not a very common one at that since it was most appropriate when the patient was unconscious and otherwise unable to respond. More common would be the "guidance-cooperation" model, which was described as equivalent to parent-child interaction in which the former gave direction and the latter obeyed. Most prevalent, however, was the "mutual participation" model of cooperation and mutual trust between doctor and patient. This served to extend the range of behavior in the relationship.

Another extension of Parsons' concept was provided by Bloom (1965), whose model incorporated sociocultural factors such as kinship and professional reference groups as important influences on the relationship. Thus, the exchange between physician and patient in the sick role was influenced by membership in kinship, ethnic, and other reference groups for the patient and membership in professional societies and other subcultural reference groups for the physician. This analysis served to broaden the context in which the interaction took place.

A quite different criticism is illustrated by the approach taken by Freidson (1961) among others. The underlying theoretical assumptions are based on conflict theory, rather than the structural-functionalist approach of Parsons. Conflict theory engenders a different perspective of the role of deviant behavior (e.g., deviance may be a source of desirable change in the system and not necessarily something to be corrected). Thus, the sick role, which from the functionalist perspective is seen as a way to control and limit deviance, would be seen as dysfunctional from a conflict theorist's perspective because it would limit the potential for social change. Freidson goes on to challenge the assertion that the doctor-patient relationship would operate despite the differences in status and power. Situational effects and organizational contexts that were mostly ignored by Parsons take on major importance in shaping the nature of the interaction around the sick role. Here such issues as type of organizational setting, work norms, and processes such as labeling of patients and stigmatization based on degree and type of illness become operative in the failure of professional controls to prevent potential social, psychological, and economic exploitation of the patient. Unmet expectations on the parts of both doctor and patient could exacerbate the loss of mutual respect and trust necessary to the effectiveness of a relationship that is asymmetrical in power and status. More recently, conflict theory was extended in Marxist terms: the maintenance of illness in the population was described as necessary for profit by the medical profession and the health care businesses that support it (Health PAC, 1970).

A Marxist's critique claims that a mechanistic view of the human organism is promoted by medicine and the specialized capitalist organizations that undergird it because this permits the profession to see disease and disability as problems of individual patients and not of illness-generating factors in the social environment. Furthermore, the esoteric knowledge of medicine provides a special status with the right to exert control over others and the power to exploit others for profit (Waitzkin, 1978), while the "medicalization of deviance" continues to expand physicians' control (Zola, 1975).

A somewhat different approach was taken by Illich in describing medical care in general and the medical profession in particular as being iatrogenic at three levels: clinical iatrogenesis involves a lack of knowledge and errors in judgment; social iatrogenesis involves unnecessarily keeping patients in the sick role and inhibiting full participation in their social systems; and structural iatrogenesis destroys the motivation of people to take responsibility for their own problems (Illich, 1975). Other writers have adopted a more moderate tone, but the excessive autonomy of physicians, the failure of collegial controls, and the vulnerability of the patient in the sick role to exploitation remain as principal themes (Waitzkin & Waterman, 1974).

The final item in this selective review and the most recent is a critique by Gallagher (1976). In the main, his criticisms of the Parsonian conceptualization are:

1. the illness as deviance conception fails to account for behaviors associated with chronic disease or disability,
2. it cannot account for health maintenance behavior (or preventive medicine, in general), and
3. the concept does not adequately account for variations in physician behavior in different organizational settings. Moreover, Parsons' concept is "medico-centric in that it overestimates the capabilities of physicians and underestimates the importance of family and community resources in coping with ill health.

Looking back over the 25 or so years, the theoretical framework of the sick role and the doctor-patient interaction has evolved considerably. Special note should be made of the redefinition of disease in terms of a less reductionistic model and of illness as a problem of adjustment rather than solely as nonnegligent deviant behavior. Also, the physician has become more of a manager than agent of control. This does permit consideration of chronic conditions and disabilities along with changes in behavior of people with respect to the value of "good health" (e.g., trends in exercise, dieting, smoking cessation). Change in the attributes of the sick role in the light of the evolving situational context of health care delivery is less clear. Some progress in clarification is possible, however, because Parsons' original formulation stimulated a great deal of research.

Tests of the Functionalist Model

Alexander Segall (1976a) recently published a review of two decdes of research on the sick role in which he made four major points. First, and perhaps most obvious, the characteristics of the sick role did not adequately describe the situation of the psychiatrically ill. Among others, he cites Petroni's (1972) review, and concludes that the"medical and psychiatric sick role models entail rather different types of reciprocal relationship between doctor and patient."

Second, the expectations of the sick role vary widely depending upon the illness, especially for chronic diseases. For example, it was pointed out that: ". . . chronic illness by definition is not temporary. Consequently role expectations that one should try to get well, overcome the condition and resume functioning in a (normal pre-illness) capacity are inappropriate" (Kassebaum & Bauman, 1965). A similar point was made regarding the status of the aged, especially in the case of terminal illness, for which a "terminal sick role" variation was proposed (Lipman & Sterne, 1965).

Third, research findings showed wide sociocultural variations in perception of the rights and obligations of the sick role. One example is Twaddle's (1969) study of a small sample in which only a minority perceived the elements of the sick role in a manner consistent with Parsons' model. Later replications tended also to raise questions about the adequacy of the sick role as originally postulated (Bercanovic, 1972).

Fourth, willingness to adopt the sick role has been the subject of extensive research efforts. The findings do suggest that there is a wide range of factors that can influence this particular element of the sick role. However, Segall believed that both conceptual and methodological problems have precluded an adequate test of the concept.

Since publication of that survey, Segall (1976b) has reported on a study of his own, which tested expectations of the sick role of hospitalized patients and whether sociocultural differences existed in two groups of patients regarding willingness to adopt the sick role. Few differences between the groups were found, although there was agreement that illness was an undesirable state and that people should be motivated to be healthy.

On a more positive note, a recent study tended to support the validity of Parsons' original concept. A survey of nearly 500 discharged patients reported agreement with each of the sick role expectations, although there was no correlation among them (Arluke, Kennedy, & Kessler, 1979). The duty to get well was most strongly supported by young, educated females living alone. The duty to seek professional help was widely accepted, but did not vary by any characteristic except age. Older patients were more likely to agree than younger ones. Not being responsible for illness was an expectation most strongly held by older respondents and those with low incomes. Finally, almost everyone agreed that the sick person should be exempt from normal roles. It should also be noted that none of the predictor equations accounted for much of the variance. Nonetheless, the authors concluded: ". . . when the expectations are considered discretely, the Parsons model is a fairly accurate descriptor of major patterns of sick role expectations in our data" (Arluke, Kennedy, & Kessler, (1979:35).

Tests of the Conflict Model

It was suggested earlier that there is an alternative theoretical approach to the sick role—that provided by conflict theory. Broadly speaking, three major themes emerge from proponents of this perspective. First, there is a rigid stratification system in medicine: among physicians, between physicians and other health practitioners, and, especially, between doctors and patients. Second, illness is seen as a source of exploitation in exposing the vulnerable sick person to physicians (and others) who occupy superordinate positions. A third theme concerns the companies that support the medical profession (e.g., professional societies, medical institutions, pharmaceutical manufacturers) in exploiting others for profit (Waitzkin & Waterman, 1974). Of these themes, only the first two are directly relevant to the topic here.

Empirical studies of the sick role that stem from the conflict model are much less common in literature. An important exception, of course, is the work of Eliot Freidson, whose research on medicine and medical care has received wide attention. Although his critiques have ranged broadly, he has most recently concentrated on issues of stratification in medicine and the consequences of unchecked professional autonomy (Freidson, 1970a; 1970c). In his most recent work (Freidson, 1975) he showed clearly that collegial controls are inadequate to ensure the expression of a "collectivity orientation" and a high quality of care in actual practice.

The effects on communication of inequality in status of doctor and patient have also been studied. A report of a pretest of a study of communication patterns between doctor and patient suggested that how much and the manner in which information was communicated formed a basis for assessment of physician uncertainty and power relationships in the interaction (Waitzkin & Stoeckle, 1976). Another report indicated that despite the importance to patients of information about their illnesses, their passivity in the interaction with physicians left control of how much knowledge was gained to the latter (Boreham & Gibson, 1978). Danziger (1978), however, showed that some negotiation can occur despite unequal status, depending upon how active or passive the patient played her role and whether the doctor's role was more of an "expert, a counselor or co-participant." Other factors that have been found to foster the functioning of the doctor-patient relationship despite status and power differences include past successful treatment (Caterinicchio, 1979), the physician's willingness to express a caring attitude and to explain the medical condition (DiMatteo, Prince & Taranta, 1979), and biomedical innovation (Sorenson, 1974). This last is interesting in that the author found that routine medical encounters involved high professional control and the corollary, high patient dependency. Biomedical innovations, such as new drugs, often resulted in a higher degree of professional uncertainty and increased willingness to communicate with patients. This reduced the degree of professional control and increased the discretionary power of the patient. Finally, but not exhaustively, in a cross-cultural context, Krause (1977) noted that where medicine is a not-for-profit occupation, there is no exploitation of the patient despite differences in knowledge and expertise because the patient is not viewed as inferior to the physician.

The latent functions of illness have received considerable reinterpretation but little empirical study by functionalists and conflict theorists alike. An exception was an early project by Shuval (1970), which attempted to explain very high rates of utilization of physician services by different groups of Israelis that could not be explained by levels of morbidity. Some findings that were called "latent functions" included need for social contact (Parsons' "secondary gain"), coping with failure, and a mechanism for integration of immigrants into Israeli society. Waitzkin (1971) illustrated the latent function of the sick role as a means of control of deviant behavior in various institutional settings such as mental hospitals, prisons, and military units. And Gerson (1976) has recently concluded that illness as deviance is inadequate to explain sick role behavior because illness is simultaneously the physician's work and the disabling of the patient's self. Rather, he suggests that illness should be seen as political process, permitting a more realistic evaluation of the realities of doctor-patient interaction and the organizational complexity of contemporary medical settings.

The apparent differences between the functionalists and conflict theorists in conceptualization of the sick role have been somewhat reconciled in a recent statement by Renee Fox (1977) in which she outlines some issues emerging from the processes of "medicalization and demedicalization of society." While acknowledging modification of the original sick role concept, she still finds it central to understanding the consequences of the process of "medicalization of deviance," which places more and more responsibility and authority in the hands of physicians and increases the powerlessness of the sick person. The reaction to this trend is "demedicalization," an attempt to destratify the doctor-patient relationship. Some indicators of this are official statements of "patient's rights" that are part of the code of hospital care; substituting the term "consumer" for "patient"; urging the licensing of nurse practitioners and other doctor-alternates, both as a symbolic reduction of physician autonomy and as a practical matter. Perhaps most current is the emphasis on self-care and engaging in "healthful behavior." Fox suggests that: ". . . the underlying assumption in these instances is that . . . not only will persons with a medical problem be free from some of the exigencies of the sick role, but both personal and public health will thereby improve, all with considerable savings in cost" (1977:99). After further analysis, she concludes that demedicalization will indeed alter some facets of the sick role, but the effects will be limited because:

> . . . the shifts in emphasis from illness to health, from therapeutic to preventive medicine, and from the dominance and autonomy of the doctor to patients' rights and greater control of the medical profession do not alter the fact that health and illness and medicine are the central preoccupations in the society which have diffuse symbolic as well as practical meaning.[Fox, 1977:21]

Sick Role and the Elderly

The special situation of the elderly with respect to their devalued status, high levels of social and health needs, and lower levels of resources have been sufficiently described and need not be repeated here (Shanas & Maddox, 1976). However, despite the increased research effort on aging and the aged, relatively little attention has been paid to the aged and the sick role. In this respect, there are at least four areas in which general considerations of the sick role may affect the elderly more profoundly if not differently from the effects on younger people. First, status differences between doctor and patient may be exacerbated because of lower levels of educational achievement by today's elderly and their greater unfamiliarity with advances in modern medical technology, Second, a high proportion of older persons today maintain beliefs and values derived from ethnic subcultures. These may not always be compatible with the ideology of modern medical practice relative to when to seek professional help or to comply with treatment regimens.

Third, status and cultural differences may relate to an uncritical assumption by elderly patients that the physician is fully competent and an expectation that the physician will exhibit a more personal interest in the patient's problems (Linn, 1975). Finally, but not exhaustively, the relative ineffectiveness of modern medicine with chronic disease raises questions anew about the viability of the acute-care-oriented medical model, and opens medical practitioners and support organizations to the charges of exploiting illness in the elderly for personal gain.

Much of the research that has been done on elderly subjects relates either to perceptions of the sick role or to factors leading to adopting the sick role. Illustrative of the first is a study of the impact of Medicare on the sick role (Coe & Peterson, 1973). It was hypothesized that Medicare, defined as an innovation in mechanisms for payment of services, would lead to a redefinition by the elderly of the meaning of symptoms and a subsequent increased utilization of physicians, and that this would result in emergence of a "non-deviant sick role." The results of the study, conducted between 1965 and 1971 by means of household surveys, showed that symptoms were redefined from being "normal conditions of aging" to being indicators of illness and that rates of utilization of physicians did increase. However, there was no evidence of perception of a nondeviant sick role associated with chronic diseases. Role expectations based on characteristics of acute illnesses like those of Parsons' original model were maintained.

More recently, in a study of institutionalized elderly, hypotheses concerning the effects of total institutions on a tendency to define oneself as sick and to play the sick role were not supported. In fact, it was found that these institutionalized elderly were less likely to incorporate the illness label into their definition of self (Myles, 1978). Finally, a recent study reported that older patients were more likely than younger ones to accept the subordinate and dependent role of patient and less likely to challenge the doctor's authority. This may be an effect of lower level of consumer sophistication and culturally induced inhibitions for challenging authority found among the current elderly. It was suggested that this may change as the current cohort of younger patients becomes older (Haug, 1979).

Willingness to adopt the sick role by the elderly has been more extensively examined, but the results vary widely and do not lead to easy summarization. Some studies report that the elderly are slower to adopt the sick role than younger people even for life-threatening conditions because of multiple and pervasive symptoms. That is, even symptoms of a heart attack were not viewed by the elderly in an "illness context." Previous experience with symptoms, availability of medication used before, and a reluctance to "bother" the doctor with symptoms that may go away all served to delay seeking care for a potentially fatal attack (Alonzo, 1977). Others have focused on situational factors, and suggest that having access to a regular source of care is more important than perceived illness in willingness to define oneself as sick (Wan, n.d.). Another emphasis is on the elderly person's perception of the physician's role. In one national survey, fewer elderly than younger respondents reported having confidence in the capability of organized medicine (not necessarily in their private doctor); confidence was lowest among the elderly poor (Kleinman & Clemente, 1976). Despite these reservations, adopting the sick role by the elderly was facilitated by perception of the physician as having a personal interest in the patient. The influence was particularly strong when the patient had an accessible, regular source of care (Nuttbrock & Kosberg, 1978). Clearly, we have much to learn about both the concept and its behavioral components with respect to the elderly.

Retrospect and Prospect

Parsons' concept of the sick role has had remarkable endurance and a pervasive influence in the more than quarter century since formal publication. We have reviewed examples of research that attempted to test its components. In general, results provide very little direct support for the expectations or their expression in behavior. Much of this research and the conceptual criticisms suggest many areas of needed expansion of the concept —illness as nondeviance, control as a facet of management that allows for negotiation on a more egalitarian basis, etc. Almost all critics have called for much more investigation of the range of illness behavior and health behavior.

Perhaps the question should be asked: can there be a *new* concept of the sick role that will more adequately and completely explain the range of observed behavior if the underlying assumptions of the medical model remain? The reductionist nature of the medical model and its limited ability to extend understanding of the sick role behavior, especially among the elderly, has been described by Engel (1977b). However, even his proposed addition of a psychosocial dimension to the biomedical perspective only extends the bases on which a reductionist theory is built. The "fault" for illness still is external to the individual. The recent emphasis on life-style as a source of disease development in late life has led to formulation of a "voluntaristic" model of disease. Although Veatch (1980) questions whether life-style behaviors associated with health risks are truly voluntary, the voluntaristic model does raise the possiblity for developing a concept of sick role behavior that includes both externally and internally derived causes of disease. This, in turn, may alter the concept of deviance and its application to the sick role as a means of control.

Antonovsky (1979) has recently proposed a different conceptual approach, one that rejects the assumptions commonly associated with the pathogenic model and substitutes those associated with what he calls "salutogenesis." The model is far too complex to describe here; but it is noteworthy that it introduces new elements such as a "sense of coherence" and has redefined older ones such as stress, resistance resources, and tension management as part of a "Health Ease-Dis-ease Continuum." Most of all, physical, biological, and behavioral factors are united into a complex but integrated conceptual model that focuses on questions about how people stay healthy. Such a perspective not only rejects the notion of illness as deviance, but postulates a very different role for healers. That is, the social and physical environment is seen as inherently stressful, and positions toward the "dis-ease" end of the continuum would be expected. In fact, the majority of people in any population are found toward the "ease" end of the continuum. The question, then, is not what makes people dis-eased, but how do they maintain ease? Attention is focused on coping behaviors rather than control of deviance. Likewise, health personnel are viewed as one of many potential general resistance resources, and should perform as orchestrators of maximizing ability of clients to resist stress-induced dis-ease. Other implications for the sick role beg to be explored.

The salutogenic model may be worthy of such exploration for clarification of the aged person and the sick role as well as for the many other facets that the model suggests. Because of the influence of culture on definitions of health and illness, there ought to be more emphasis on cross-cultural investigations. Finally, we have been concerned in this chapter with the aged. Certainly, emphasis on the special situation of the health of the elderly in future research is also to be encouraged.

PART II

BARRIERS TO
DOCTOR–ELDERLY PATIENT
RELATIONSHIPS

Defining the problem is the preliminary intellectual task critical to working out possible solutions. This section undertakes to define the problematic issues in relationships between doctors and elderly patients using three perspectives: that of physician, older person, and gerontologist. Each considers obstacles to a successful relationship or even establishing a relationship in the first place, and not surprisingly, their viewpoints converge. The practicing specialist in geriatric medicine, Dr. Williams, identifies three types of obstacles, those within the physician, those within the patient, and those within the environment. He makes a significant point, that treating older patients is the most complicated form of medical practice, yet medical students, residents, and physicians in the field in the main are not being given and do not have the necessary training, knowledge, or experience to deal with the health needs of the elderly. As a consequence, practitioners may be as subject to "ageism" as the general public. Isaac Fine, who gives the patient viewpoint, also alludes to inadequate knowledge, but not only that of the physician. He notes the need for *new* knowledge, to be gained by research, so as to provide medicine with new tools for treating the ills that the elderly are heir to. He also makes a plea for the transmission from doctor to patient of knowledge and more explanations of the reasons for recommended treatments and the characteristics of prescribed medicine.

Williams recognizes the inadequacies of present forms of financing through Medicare and Medicaid. Fine adds to this the complexity of the payment system, with confusing multiple types of paperwork, and the bewildering array of services and requirements. He recommends political action to secure adoption of a comprehensive health care system to correct a situation in which, as Fine so aptly puts it, "a high technology product is delivered by a cottage industry structure."

Dr. Ethel Shanas, the gerontologist, concurs on the financial obstacles suffered by the elderly in the quest for good health care. In general, she bases her presentation on empirical data secured from surveys of older persons, among whom about a million report need for care, but are failing to seek it for monetary reasons. Shanas also stresses further a point made by the others, namely that some elderly consider their complaints are due to old age rather than illness, and are not worth "bothering" a doctor with. She thus touches on, but does not develop, a possibly significant issue: the *status* differences between the prestigious physician and the denigrated old person, which lead to feelings that the mere fact of seeking the services that the practitioner is there to give is somehow pestering him. This undoubtedly links with another point made by Shanas: that older patients need more time for a visit because of their multiple ailments, while time is a scarce commodity for most physicians. An added obstacle is the difficulty the elderly face in getting to the doctor. In an era when home visits are the rare exceptions, lack of transportation can prevent office visits, to which Williams adds the physical barriers in physicians' office buildings as another environmental deterrent.

Qualities that apply to the interaction between physicians and the elderly, once they get together, as distinct from the hurdles involved in reaching that point, also are noted by all three contributors. Included are both physician and patient chracteristics, such as a lack of knowledge, fearful attitudes, and failures in communication. Fragmentation of services and discontinuity of care, while not discussed here, are important to consider. An older person who needs to see a variety of specialists may not have any one general practitioner or family physician to coordinate care; as a result, there is no opportunity to build up the mutual trust and understanding essential for quality care and a satisfying relationship.

An explicit definition is needed of what constitutes a *successful* doctor-elderly patient relationship, as the criterion against which obstacles to that relationship should be measured. What is actually being impeded? Although the contributors do not say directly, all three imply at least two facets of a successful relationship: satisfaction with the encounter on the part of both parties, and achievement of the purpose of the encounter, be it prevention, therapy, reassurance, or simply empathic understanding, These assumptions lie beneath the surface not only in the chapters presented here, but also in the chapters that follow, especially in Chapter 9, by Victor Marshall.

One common theme emerges from the chapters in this section, however. In defining the problem, that is, identifying obstacles to a successful doctor-patient relationship when the patient is elderly, one must consider characteristics of the physician, of the patient, and also of the environment in which interaction occurs.

3
The Viewpoint of a Gerontologist

ETHEL SHANAS, Ph.D.

Introduction

The barriers to a doctor-patient relationship can be considered from two points of view: that of the doctor and that of the patient. In this chapter, older people speak for themselves on this topic through their responses to relevant questions in national sample surveys, and then I give my own interpretation of what barriers seem to keep the physician from successfully communicating with his older patient. I first report on the general state of health of older people in the United States and the use of physicians both by people who feel their health is good and by people who feel their health is poor. Then I summarize some of the reasons why older people do not see doctors. Finally, I try to present the barriers to a doctor-patient relationship from the point of view of the physician as I perceive it.

How the Elderly View their Health

The reports on health status of the elderly and their use of physicians come from nationwide probability studies of noninstitutionalized persons aged 65 and over. In studies such as these, there are no volunteer subjects. The respondents are preselected to represent the elderly population of the United States. In this discussion, one may assume that the respondents in these surveys represent the total population of the United States aged 65 and over living outside of institutions. At any one time, only about 5 percent of the elderly are in institutions; thus, these studies may be thought of as a snapshot of the majority of the elderly, the other 95 percent.

In the United States most persons aged 65 and over are well, not sick. In 1975, about 5 of every 10 old persons interviewed said without further qualification that their health was good. About 2 of every 10 described their health as poor. In between these two groups were people who said their health was fair or who described limitations in their health status. These people, however, did not say their health was poor. Despite this optimistic view of their health by the elderly, substantial numbers of older people see physicians. In 1975, about one-third of all older people, some 8 million persons, said they saw a physician in the month before they were interviewed. In any typical month, then, physicians see about one-third of the community-resident elderly, either in their offices, in clinics, or in the hospital. Many internists tell us that all of their patients are elderly. Given the data just reported here, this may indeed be true.

Let us consider the use of medical care by the elderly, first by those who say their health is good and then by those who say their health is poor. Among those old people who said their health was good, 1 of every 4 had seen a doctor during the previous month. One may well ask: if people feel their health is good, why have they seen a doctor? I will answer this rhetorical question by quoting from a pioneer in the study of diseases of old age, Dr. Robert T. Monroe. Dr. Monroe was a teacher at Harvard. He was an internist who saw older people as total persons, not only as organ systems. Drawing on his observations in clinical practice, he said: "Old people have more than the young to be sick with and to be sick of, yet they call themselves well if they view their balance as satisfactory and sick when they find it less than so." Dr. Monroe's comments help explain why one-fourth of those persons who described their health as good saw a doctor during the previous month. These people were functioning well. As Dr. Monroe would have said, they feel themselves well because their balance is well. Nevertheless, they have pathology that brings them to the doctor. Many of them had the chronic illnesses of old age, heart complaints, diabetes, arthritis, that doctors see in their practice. However, these persons did not see themselves as in need of such services as sheltered care, meals on wheels, or special services. All these are services that some segments of the elderly populaion need desperately, but not these elderly persons who think their health is good.

Those elderly who said their health was poor and who saw doctors are a minority of the aged, but a minority with a great many needs. Their needs encompass not only medical care from a physician, but many other kinds of services. People who say they are in poor health are far more likely than other older people to be housebound. They are far more likely to be mobile with difficulty. Vertigo is an extremely common ailment among these people. Half of these persons report that they experienced vertigo, that they were dizzy during the previous week. These older people say that they are afraid to go out and afraid that they are going to fall.

About 2 percent of the American population over the age of 65, most of whom said their health was poor, said that they fell during the week before they were interviewed. This is almost half a million persons among a population of some 23 million people. Dizziness and vertigo are terrifying experiences. Let me illustrate. I visited an apartment house in which many of the tenants were older people. One of the women I spoke to said, "The lady upstairs worries me." My respondent was herself a woman in her eighties living alone, the lady upstairs was 2 years older. "Why does she worry you?" I asked. "Well, she cannot walk straight," she replied. She then pointed out to me, through her window, her neighbor doing her shopping. The neighbor needed to have her own gyroscope. She was dizzy, going from one edge of the sidewalk to another, and she was going to the grocery store. I was terrified that she was going to fall because could not walk straight. I asked my respondent why her neighbor was outside by herself. "Well," she said, "she doesn't have anyone to shop for her. She doesn't have any children."

Patients' Barriers to Treatment

While about one-third of all elderly persons, 8 million people, said they saw a doctor during the month before they were interviewed in 1975, about 13 percent of the elderly, that is about 3 million people, said they needed medical care or treatment, but they delayed or put off such care or treatment. What were the barriers to older people consulting a doctor?

The first barrier was lack of money. When Title XVIII of the Social Security Act, the so-called Medicare amendment, was enacted in 1965, it was expected that it would relieve the financial burden of medical care costs of the elderly. In 1975, however, 4 percent of all elderly in the United States, almost a million persons, said they postponed medical care and treatment because they did not have the money for such care. In 1957, in a somewhat similar study, this same question was asked: "Is there anything about your health that has not been taken care of? Why?" At that time, well before Medicare, about the same proportion of the elderly, roughly 4 percent, said lack of money was the reason for their not seeking medical care. What is important here is that there are now almost a million elderly people in this country who say, "Yes, there is something that bothers me. Yes, I do have a problem, but I am not going to see a doctor because I do not have the money."

Other reasons given by older people in 1975 for not seeking medical care were similar to responses made by such persons 20 years earlier. One standard reason is, "I'm not sick enough to see a doctor." It is difficult to know the auspicious moment to see a doctor. The American population, elderly or not, is confused by propaganda that urges self-care of health and no wasting of doctors' time. One is supposed to know when to take care of one's health, when not to waste the doctor's time, and when, at the appropriate moment, to see the doctor. One of the major reasons why people do not see a doctor, then, is that they do not think they are "sick enough." At the same time, these people have told us that there is a health problem, a physical problem that bothers them and that they think requires care or treatment.

Another reason often given for not seeing a doctor, and again it is one that is as common now as it was 20 years ago, is "What can the doctor do for me?" Many people who are over 65 believe that aches and pains are a usual part of old age. The beliefs of these respondents do not differ greatly from those held by many professionals. The answer "What can the doctor do for me?" perhaps reflects the thinking, "It is just old age, and I am just going to be a bother to the doctor if I see him."

In addition to lack of money, feelings that the respondent was not yet sick enough for the doctor, and feeling that the doctor could not help, there was a new reason given in 1975 for not seeking care or treatment of health problems. This was the difficulty respondents had getting to the doctor. Home visits to the elderly by physicians in the United States have become less and less common. Only about 4 percent of all elderly persons in this country, something less than a million people, reported that they had home calls from physicians when they were ill during the previous year. Many of the 3 million persons who said they had extended health problems also said: "I would have gone to the doctor, but I can't get there." And, apparently, the doctor cannot get to them.

The patient's barriers to a doctor-patient relationship fall into two major categories, one of these categories encompasses externals that can be remedied, such as lack of money or lack of transportation. The second of these categories is people's attitude. As long as older people feel that the physician cannot help them, as long as there are programs of public education that give conflicting signals to people such as "take care of your health and do not bother the doctor and see the doctor if you feel sick," as long as older people say of their ailments "it's old age," there will continue to be patient barriers to patient-doctor relationships.

Physicians' Barriers to Treatment

Let us now consider some of the barriers to doctor-patient relationships from the physician's point of view. Some years ago, Dr. Irvine H. Page of the Cleveland Clinic published a statement on medical education. What he said in 1968 is still relevant and helpful in understanding physician attitudes towards elderly patients. "To an important degree," said Dr. Page, "the future physician depends on the imprinting he receives in his medical school experience." Although there are many innovative changes underway in medical education, the current emphases in the training of the student physician and, certainly, the past emphases in the training of many practicing physicians bear little relationship to the needs of the older patient. Medical education stresses treatment and cure. The older patient has chronic conditions and other ailments for which cure is sometimes impossible. Many physicians are discouraged about elderly patients before they begin their treatment. The"what-can-you-expect-at-your-age" syndrome that the physician may feel is communicated to the patient. Many times, too, the physician feels threatened by his elderly patients because he cannot cure them. For such doctors, elderly patients are a pain, a psychological pain, because the doctor feels frustrated by his inability to help them.

Another barrier to doctor-patient relationships is that physicians do not have the time to give elderly patients. The National Center for Health Statistics has collected data from physicians on the age of their patients, the presenting complaints, how much time the doctor gave the patient, and what treatment they gave the patient. The average time given to the average patient aged 65 and over is 15 minutes. The older patient is likely to be less medically sophisticated than the younger patient, may have multiple complaints, and may neglect to mention complaints because they are embarrassing or because he or she thinks they may be trivial. The physician who treats the elderly must be prepared for all of these contingencies. It is difficult to tell busy doctors to allow more time for their elderly patients, but such time allowance is essential for there to be effective doctor-patient communication.

Finally, the relationship of the physician to the family of the older person may be a barrier to communication between doctor and patient. Many times the older person comes to the physician's office with a family member. Here the doctor must encourage the patient to speak for himself or herself. But whether the older person is alone or with a family member, in the office, hospital, or at home, the physician treating the older person has to work with the family of that person. If a health regimen is to be followed, if proper care is to be given, the family must be informed of the patient's medical problem and of how they can help in its treatment.

A Look Ahead

I look forward to a resolution of the barriers in doctor-patient relationships as they affect the aging patient. With ongoing changes in medical education, physicians are becoming more sophisticated about older patients as people. They are learning how to listen, they are becoming more tolerant of their aged patient, "our future selves" as the National Institute on Aging describes them. As older people become more educated and more sophisticated, they in turn are better able to communicate with doctors and to tell the doctor what ails them in terms he or she can understand. The physician must realize that older people are not merely organ systems, that their problems may be social as well as medical. The elderly patient, in turn, must be educated to realize that physicians are not God.

4

The Physician Viewpoint

T. Franklin Williams, M.D.

Physicians working with older patients—and this includes most physicians —face obstacles of at least three general types in achieving good relationships with these patients and providing the desired care. These three types of obstacles are those found within the physician himself or herself, those found within the patient, and those related to limitations in resources and the environment. Of these, I will give most attention to the obstacles that exist within physicians themselves.

Physician-Generated Barriers

Physicians have trouble working effectively with older people because of limitations in their own knowledge, experience or skills, and attitudes related to aging. In terms of knowledge, most physicians in practice today receive little or no instruction about the nature of aging and the special constellation of disabilities that commonly affect the elderly. The average physician has the same misconceptions about aging as the general public. These are some common misconceptions: that there is inevitable physical failing, inevitable mental failing, inevitable sexual failing, that most elderly are in institutions, most are separated from families, most want to live with families, and most want to withdraw. All of these myths have been dispelled by adequate studies. I will not dwell on them in any detail except to point out that in one of the areas, physical failing, data taken from Dr. Nathan Schock's work at the Baltimore Gerontological Research Center of the National Institute of Aging shows that with normal aging decline in organ function is never complete or really very extreme because of all the reserves we all have in our body functions: the amount remaining in every organ system is more than enough for any ordinary activity. In fact, physical decline with age, although definite, is relatively modest in relation to what is needed for day to day activities. The same can be shown for mental failing, sexual failing, and the like.

It is most important that physicians understand that aging itself is a relatively benign affair, *if* the older person is fortunate enough not to acquire severe chronic diseases and disabilities. Yet, all too often, patients will tell how a physician has said, in response to description of a symptom, "What do you expect at your age?" or "This must be due to your age, and there is nothing we can do about it." Sir Ferguson Anderson, the great geriatrician of Glasgow, tells of how one man in his eighties handled such a physician's comment when the man went to the physician about a pain in his right knee. When told that it was because of his age, the man said, "But doctor, my left knee is the same age as my right, and it's not hurting."

The second area of knowledge needed by physicians in dealing with the elderly concerns the constellation of health-related problems that are different from those commonly seen among younger patients and until now inadequately addressed in medical education. Major differences are apparent in the ways illness affects elderly people compared to nonelderly. A striking example of the difference in presenting complaints for elderly was illustrated for me on a visit to a general hospital in Australia in which there was a special geriatric ward, to which were admitted all persons over age 75. One result of this admitting practice was that it was easy to see, collected there on one ward, what were the common presenting causes for hospital admission among the elderly. Half the patients on the ward the day I visited had come to the hospital as a result of a fall. Data from a study of an elderly population in England confirmed the high frequency. Exton-Smith (1977) shows in one survey that the frequency of falls rises from age 65 almost continuously on to age 85. There is a slight dip in males in the oldest age groups, which is not completely explained, but overall the annual incidences are running at a 50 percent level in women beyond the age of 80 or 85. Thus, the differential diagnosis of falling among elderly is obviously important, a differential diagnosis that would rarely arise in younger people.

Another common presenting complaint by elderly persons or, more often, by family members is that of failing mental function—again, a rare complaint in younger people. Here again, unfortunately, many physicians are not aware of the advances being made in basic understanding about causes of dementia in the elderly. It appears quite clear, as already noted, that mental function declines relatively little as a result of aging itself, and one or another specific pathological process produces dementia when it does become an evident problem for an elderly person. It is very important that we be as precise as possible in prescription because in at least a few instances successful treatment is possible. We may reasonably expect to have increased understanding of causes and potential treatments within the next few years. In relation to this, we have to pay particular attention to the frequency with which depression is masked as dementia.

In relation to the second difference in treatment of older patients, the need to deal with multiple chronic disabilities simultaneously, almost all elderly persons unfortunately do acquire several chronic diseases or disabilities, as well as face almost inevitable psychosocial burdens in the form of losses of spouse, friends, job, income. The treatment of any one of these conditions or any new acute condition requires attention to the interacting effects among the various other problems. Here the applicability of the Engel biopsychosocial model is especially noteworthy. Taking care of older patients is the most complicated form of medical practice and success at it has been called the "fruition of the clinicians."

The third type of knowledge of disease a physician needs to work effectively with the elderly is an understanding of the importance of even small gains in function, or stabilization of function, for a disabled elderly person. For example, the ability to transfer independently from bed to wheelchair for an elderly person with a stroke may make all the difference between whether he or she can get along at home with limited family help or will need to enter a nursing home.

Finally, in this list of special types of knowledge needed by physicians, is the knowledge and experience to deal with a special type of crisis faced by most older people at one time or another and very rarely by younger people, namely, the question of whether they must leave their usual home setting to enter a nursing home or some other type of long-term care institutional setting. To be truly helpful at such times, a physician needs to be able to make medical and functional assessments that give special attention to the factors that are going to determine the patient's needs for services from others. He or she also must be able to work effectively with specially trained nurses and social workers in understanding the capabilities of the family, the home situation, and various levels of institutional care to meet the needs of this particular patient. Studies that we have done in Rochester have shown quite clearly that such a comprehensive evaluation process and assistance in appropriate decision making can make a major difference in what happens to old people.

To go on to consider other areas of obstacles in the physician to his working with the elderly, that of lack of experience is closely related, of course, to the lack of knowledge. I am thinking specifically of the average physician's lack of experience in his or her training in caring for elderly patients in settings where their needs were receiving special emphasis, and the lack of teachers who were especially interested in the elderly who could guide this experience. One approach to remedying this deficiency is the one we are taking at the University of Rochester, where students and house staff have clinical experiences at Monroe Community Hospital, a setting devoted explicitly to the care of elderly and chronically ill people. The house staff and students almost invariably report, at the end of a rotation with us, that they have acquired a different perspective on care of the elderly from what they had learned in the ordinary acute hospital or clinic setting. The report of the special committee of the Institute of Medicine of the National Academy of Sciences on the teaching of aging in medical education (Institute of Medicine, 1978), in addition to calling for more explicit aging-related content in essentially all courses in medical school, also called for learning experiences in every type of setting in which older people need care.

Finally, in terms of the physician's own characteristics that may present obstacles to effective relationships with elderly persons, is the matter of the physician's own attitude toward aging and elderly people. In my view, much of this attitude is related to the matters already discussed, namely, lack of knowledge and lack of experience. I have seen many house officers, who came to Monroe Community Hospital quite skeptical about the value of this rotation for them, who find that the satisfactions of helping older people make small but very important gains in function and the satisfactions of participating in successful arrangements for home support services produce a new and favorable outlook on caring for older patients. I see the continued strengthening of knowledge and experience in caring for the elderly as the single most effective approach we have to change the commonly negative attitudes toward elderly patients that many physicians have. Overall, it appears that physicians share the general society's "ageism," and although physicians may be expected to help take the lead in changing such views, the changes are going to be necessary throughout society before physicians as well as others will be freed from their biases, fears, and guilt feelings.

Patient-Generated Barriers

Turning now from physician characteristics, it is also true that some characteristics of elderly patients have a negative impact on the physician's own approach to relationships with them. Probably the most common in my experience is the tendency of elderly patients to attribute health problems and symptoms simply to old age, to think that little or nothing can be done to help, and thus to avoid or postpone consulting a physician. As I have already stated, many physicians unfortunately have reinforced just such a negative view. But the initiative really does rest in the last analysis with the patient, and until the patient goes to the physician—and, if not satisfied, goes to still another—there is no opportunity to see what contributions medical knowledge and medical practice can make.

The same problem applies in the carrying out of recommended treatment measures. Many older patients again have such a discouraged or hopeless view about their problem that they "give up" on continuing recommended therapeutic programs, particularly of such types as changes of diet and physical therapy programs. Complex issues are often involved in the problems of patient adherence to recommended regimens; here I can probably go no further than to emphasize that an ongoing physician-older patient relationship and medical care plan requires the sustained commitment of both parties to this contractual relationship between them.

Environmental Barriers

Finally, there are obstacles in the environment and in resources available for care that have an impact on the physician in his working with older patients. Most important is the need in every community for a full range of various support services and various types of institutional care settings. When these do not exist, the physician and patient are bound to be frustrated in obtaining the most appropriate type of service needed. Another type of environmental obstacle is the difficulty the older patient often faces in getting to and into the doctor's office. With the majority of older people living either in the city or in very rural areas, while physicians have been moving to the fringes of the city and suburban areas, public transportation to the doctor's office is often not available. Many office buildings still have architectural barriers for the feeble or disabled. Hospital clinics are often long distances from parking areas or bus stops and hidden in the complicated maze of large institutions.

A third major type of resource obstacle is obviously the limitation in financial resources most older people have and the limitations on the insurance payment mechanisms for health care. Any physician who has worked with older patients has had the experience numerous times of such patients avoiding their first visit to the doctor each new year because the first dollar costs have to come out of their own meager income, with Medicare Part B picking up most of the cost only after the first 60 dollars has been paid. An even more poignant common situation is that of the elderly person in need of long-term care who faces the bitter decision to use up the life savings he or she had wanted to pass on to family, and to spend down to the Medicaid level of pauperism before there will be any help in payment for long-term care, with the impoverishment of a spouse who remains at home.

In summary, physicians caring for older people face obstacles in themselves, in their older patients, and in the resources and environment with which both have to work, which are in many ways special and specific to care for older persons. Achieving better understanding of these problems should help everyone work toward their solutions.

5
The Patient Viewpoint

ISAAC FINE

The elderly feel that they owe much to the medical profession, and hold the physician in high esteem. They view the physician as an individual who is dedicated, works long hours, and is exposed to unusual hazards and stress. This esteem may be combined with the confidence that the doctor has all the answers. On balance, I think this attitude on the part of the patient is conducive to a healthy relationship with the doctor.

However, the doctor-patient relationship is no longer a one-to-one relationship. The term doctor includes general practitioners, residents, surgeons, and a wide variety of specialists, in individual or group practice. The age of the doctor might also be a consideration. The doctor is a member of certain professional organizations that have a bearing on his or her relationship with the patient.

The term elderly patient includes men and women ranging from active to frail to terminally ill; metropolitan and rural area residents; persons at various income levels; those amply covered, those inadequately covered, and those not covered by health insurance. The term patient could also include the patient's spouse or other family member. The patient also may be a member of certain organizations that have a bearing on his or her attitude towards the medical profession.

The doctor and patient meet in a variety of locations. In an office, hospital, nursing home, or perhaps even in the patient's home—the latter is now the rare exception, in light of certain cost-benefit considerations.

The initiation of the doctor-patient relationship is often based on little information on the part of the patient. The elderly patient with multiple chronic medical problems may need to start with a primary care physician. He is most likely to contact a specialist, since only 15 percent of today's physicians are general practitioners. To the extent that this is a serious mismatch, it could be a problem. Perhaps the specialist combines the services of the general practitioner with his specialty. The elderly patient displays different symptoms for the same illness. The elderly patient reacts differently to drugs than do those of lower age groups. (Incidentally, drugs are usually tested on the lower age groups.) Moreover, the patient does not know the extent of the doctor's training in geriatric medicine. Training in geriatrics equips the doctor with special knowledge, skills, and attitudes for optimum treatment of the elderly, including sensitivity to the patient's social environment. In the choice of a surgeon, the patient does not know if the surgeon is specialty board certified or not.

Quality of Care

This brings us to the consideration of the quality of care that the doctor is prepared to offer the elderly. Although almost half of today's patients are over 65, only a small percentage of doctors are trained in geriatrics. In May 1979, the National Retired Teachers Association-American Association for Retired Persons (NRTA-AARP) and the George Washington University Medical Center cosponsored a conference entitled "Geriatric Medicine —Tomorrow's Practice Today." Some 400 representatives from medical schools and teaching hospitals were in attendance. The geriatric conference was designed to give needed impetus to increased geriatric training at all levels—from medical students to practitioners. In treating the elderly, we are confronted with a skill that is in its infancy.

Continued education in geriatric medicine will make the physician especially sensitive to the weaknesses of the aged and provide early warning of potential medical problems, emotional and mental as well as physical. The need for this training is further highlighted by the fact that the over-65 population has risen from 3 million, or 4 percent of the population, in the year 1900 to more than 23 million, or 11 percent of today's population. It is estimated that the number will rise to 30 million by the year 2000.

The NRTA-AARP is represented by Joint Legislative Committees in each of the 50 states. Annually in January, some 30 members of these committees meet as a National Legislative Council in Washington to establish our legislative policies on subjects of special interest to the elderly. Our Health Policy states ". . . although issues relating to the treatment of illness dominate the discussion of health policy, the real challenge is how to maintain health and avoid illness. . . ." We regard health care as a matter of right. But there is another side to the coin, namely, the responsibility of the patient. This includes observance of a nutritionally sound diet; the observance of sound rules of personal hygiene; exercise; avoidance of excess drugs, alcohol, and tobacco; and awareness of environmental hazards, such as excess of cold or heat indoors or outdoors and taking proper precautions to guard against home accidents. Over and over again I contact a friend and find that he or she has fallen and fractured a hip. The doctor, through his staff, should reeducate the patient in the proper implementation of this responsibility. In the town of Lexington, Massachusetts, a Community Health Committee has been established with active participation by members of the local AARP chapter. This committee, working closely with the town selectmen, the Board of Health, and local doctors, has set up a course entitled "Help Yourself to Better Health with Preventive Medicine," a 10-lecture course of special interest to older persons. Incidentally, the participating physicians are serving without charge.

The Communication Gap

On the basis of an admittedly limited number of contacts, it appears to me that there is often a communication gap between doctor and patient. The doctor or a member of his staff should tell the patient why a certain drug has been prescribed and possible side effects. This could make for greater compliance. I feel I understand perfectly Mr. Glover, the case in Dr. Engel's paper. Older people have a tremendous resistance to just following instructions. They need to be told why, because when you get older you hate to admit the onset of frailty. Especially, I think, men resist this very much, and they do not want to admit that they have one condition or another. After a checkup consisting of a number of tests, the physician often tells the patient only what is wrong rather than taking the time to give the whole picture. The doctor should seriously consider establishing a communication procedure with the patient's family, especially in the case of a frail or hospitalized patient. Some 52 percent of those over 65 live with a spouse, 10 percent with other persons, 25 percent live alone, and 5 percent are in long-term care facilities. Competence should be coupled with communication. I think competence comes first. I really believe that in the case of an older person, he has to be told what this drug does and why he is taking it. Otherwise, he may just neglect to take it. Medicine is a science, but it is also an art. The science aspect is within the province of the physician. The art consists of a two-way communication between the physician and the elderly patient.

Financing

Both doctor and patient are victims of the present health care structure and method of financing medical services. There are wide gaps in the totality of medical services available to the patient. The physician as "gatekeeper" is impelled by the system to emphasize hospitalization rather than early detection and prevention. In addition, the emphasis is on long-term care facilities rather than home health care and day care.

The elderly are particularly hard hit because persons over 65 need two and a half times more medical care than the younger age groups. The per capita costs for those 65 and over in fiscal 1977 came to $1,745, compared to $661 for those 19–64, and $203 for those under 19. And as we too well know, health costs are rising at one and a half times the rate of increase of the Consumer Price Index.

This fragmented public, private, and third-party health financing system creates confusion and perplexity. The patient is asked to cope with a variety of forms, fiscal intermediaries, Medicare and Medicaid provisions, deductibles, coinsurance, covered and noncovered services, assignments accepted and assignments refused. Only 18 percent of physicians always accept Medicare assignments; 30 percent never accept them, and the balance, 52 percent, accept them only sometimes. Perhaps the complexity of the system contributes to the large percentage of doctors who do not accept assignments. Consider the bewildering collection of long-term care services and financing arrangements. At the federal level, we have the Health Care Financing Administration, the Rehabilitiation Services Administration, the Veterans Administration, the Community Services Administration, and the Administration on Aging. All, in some manner, support programs that come under the heading of long-term care.

The one-to-one relationship of the past with a simple and direct payment procedure has given way to a highly complicated procedure that has its impact on both the patient and the doctor.

Rising costs deter some elderly on a limited fixed income from seeking medical services. A number forego health care because of procedural complexities. This has led to a considerable amount of unrecognized and untreated illness among the elderly. Unrecognized hypertension and cardiac impairment might eventually entail higher costs than early treatment of such ailments. Incidentally, I have the impression that men are more apt to forego medical services because of such complexities than women. Perhaps this is one of the reasons why women outlive men.

From a financial point of view, the situation is further exacerbated by the purchase of multiple supplementary health insurance policies. The House Select Committee on Aging estimates that 4 billion dollars is spent annually for Medigap insurance and up to 1 billion dollars is spent annually on unnecessary and overlapping coverage. A number of states are doing something about this. Massachusetts now has prepared regulations to prevent the purchase of duplicated insurance and also has outlawed single-illness insurance such as cancer insurance.

Overcoming the System's Shortcomings

The complicated medical service system brings many benefits that are offset by serious shortcomings. How can the shortcomings be overcome? As stated earlier, the doctor belongs to and is influenced by professional organizations; the patient belongs to and is influenced by organizations that represent his or her interests.

This brings us to the NRTA-AARP support of the administration's efforts for health care cost containment. Legislation introduced in 1976 to cap costs at 9 percent failed to be enacted as professional medical organizations opted for voluntary controls. Legislation S570 and HR 2626, introduced in 1979, represents a continued effort at cost control.

From the long-range point of view, we support the concepts advanced before Congress and in publications by Dr. Robert N. Butler, Director of the National Institute on Aging, with respect to the need for research. According to Dr. Butler, the ultimate cost containment lies in adequate basic biomedical, clinical, and social rescaarch. Such research results in cure or prevention in place of costly care. The NRTA-AARP is represented on the National Advisory Council of the National Institute on Aging, and supports adequate appropriations for these purposes.

Regrettably, adequate funding for research is not keeping pace with the growing cost of care for chronic illnesses. In the winter 1977 issue of *Daedalus*, which was devoted to medical research, it was pointed out that it cost a billion dollars a year to take care of the victims of infantile paralysis, compared to $40 million to develop the Salk vaccine. Of course, the younger readers do not remember, but the older ones do, when TB hospitals were packed. The medical profession came up with a specific drug for the TB bacillus, and those hospitals emptied out. Going back to the issue of *Daedalus*, these outstanding investigators stated they believe that, given adequate funding, in the not-too-distant future there could be prevention or cure for cardiovascular illness, renal failure, cancer, and diabetes. I know that in Massachusetts researchers at the Joslin Clinic feel they are on the very edge of a breakthrough in regard to the prevention of diabetes.

A step in the right direction is the Health Maintenance Organization (HMO) which budgets costs, provides for capitation instead of fee-for-service, slows the pace for physicians, and places the emphasis on early detection rather than hospitalization. At the NRTA-AARP-sponsored National Legislators' Forum in October 1979, Dr. William Rox stated that the HMOs have proven conclusively they can provide the same services in a competitive system at 10 percent to 40 percent less cost than the traditional fee-for-service, cost-plus system to which the forces of the free market do not apply.

Nine states—Colorado, Connecticut, Maryland, Massachusetts, New Jersey, New York, Rhode Island, Washington, and Wisconsin—have mandatory cost-containment programs. In 1977, costs exceeded those of 1976 by 12 percent for these states, compared to a rise of 15.8 percent for the 41 states with voluntary or no programs. The National Health Planning and Resources Development Act (PL 93–641) established Health Systems Agencies with local consumer representatives. These agencies must issue Certificates of Need before additional health facilities can be built or expanded. This is another step in the right direction. In Massachusetts, the legislature is circumventing the basic purpose of this law and Certificate of need, and we are going to oppose that.

Summary

The overall picture is that of a high-technology product delivered by a cottage-industry structure. This places a strain on both patient and doctor. The structure is the problem. The NRTA-AARP believes that the Kennedy-Waxman Health Care for All Americans bill uniquely reflects our own institutions and traditions, that it provides for quality care combined with incentives for cost-saving efficiencies.

The patient looks to organizations representing the medical profession to exert their considerable influence for an effective and efficient health care delivery system, undergirded by adequate basic and clinical research. Such objectives are challenging and rewarding to the individual members of the medical profession. They reflect the individual physician's humanitarian and ethical values without impairment of a fair measure of material returns. Enactment of the Kennedy-Waxman bill would remove the barriers to and establish a healthy doctor-patient relationship.

To summarize, the barriers to a successful doctor-elderly patient relationship are, ironically, the result of progress. The life span has been extended for millions of people. Health care insurance has been provided for millions of people.

To overcome the barriers generated by these advances, tremendous new advances are necessary in the teaching and practice of geriatric medicine. This, in turn, rests on the infusion of vast sums of money into adequate funding of basic biomedical, clinical, and social research.

Finally, the delivery structure must be modernized to match the sophistication of the product, and all of this within a close personal, humane doctor-patient relationship.

Progress has always prevailed.

PART III
PATIENT CHARACTERISTICS

The previous section identified three sources of difficulties in achieving a successful doctor-elderly patient relationship: characteristics of the patients, characteristics of the physicians, and characteristics of the environment. This section explores the first of these elements, with the contributions of a gerontologist, a medical sociologist, and a psychiatrist. Alluding to aged patients' characteristics in a discussion of obstacles to success in their interaction with physicians could all too easily lead to "blaming the patient" for failures in the relationship. Fortunately, the authors of these papers do not fall into that trap. In fact, while the focus is on elderly patients, their features are analyzed against a backdrop of physician attitudes and beliefs, and it is the interplay between the two that is highlighted.

Dr. Maddox, concerned about physicians' tendencies to stereotype all the elderly as impaired, declining, and beyond help, explains in some detail the OARS method, developed at Duke University, for assessing the functional capacity of old people realistically. Contrary to the widely held negative stereotype, application of this instrument to samples in North Carolina and Ohio showed a highly differentiated group of persons over 65, in terms of social activity, economic status, mental and physical health, and activities of daily living. Most significantly, nearly 60 percent of these older persons are not functionally impaired in any of these categories, although those who are impaired are likely to suffer from multiple incapacities.

Recognition of this variability, Maddox shows, is useful not only in treatment planning and clinical management, but also in practitioner training, service staff planning, and epidemiological studies. Understanding the complexities of the elderly, physicians are less likely to be victimized by their own stereotypes and better able to deal therapeutically with their patients.

Dr. Kart examines in greater detail the stages in the definition of symptoms through which people go in trying to determine whether or not they are ill, and whether or not to seek professional care. In this process, symptoms may be attributed to external factors such as environmental stress or internal factors such as disease or biological aging. Because the elderly too often explain pain or discomfort erroneously as due to "normal aging," while the physician conveniently makes the same causal attribution, conditions that can successfully be treated or ameliorated are allowed to worsen. Thus, patient characteristics and physician stereotypes are mutually reinforcing, with negative consequences both for the relationship itself, since the patient thinks seeing the doctor is futile, and for a therapeutic outcome, since possible successful interventions are overlooked or ignored.

The theme of misattribution is carried forward by Dr. Weiss. In a series of vivid case histories from his career as a geriatric psychiatrist, he shows how patients' physical difficulties can be misinterpreted as mental problems and how mental and emotional disabilities may be misperceived as physical deterioration. Older patients who are relatively healthy but have a chronic condition are anxious and need reassurance. They may be rejected and shuffled from clinic to clinic because they are viewed as boring and cannot offer the physician evidence of therapeutic success. Weiss points out further that telling patients their symptoms are due to old age and that they should "learn to live with them" is in fact perceived by them as a message to quit bothering the doctor about something he cannot cure. Clearly, the effect on the relationship will generally be negative under these circumstances.

The title of this section might well have been "Distorted Perceptions." It is less that patient characteristics are seen as spoiling relationships with physicians than that physician stereotyping and some patients' acceptance of the stereotype pollute the relationship. However, more attention should be given to three differentiating factors among the aged, which could affect the relationship with health care providers in diverse ways. These factors are social class, race, and culture. Kart alludes to cultural variation in response to pain, and Maddox notes racial differences in functioning. However, no mention is made of the likely misperceptions of the white, generally upper-class physician who is handicapped not only by stereotypes of aging, but also by a lack of empathic understanding of the aged poor black or Spanish-speaking patient. This piles stereotype on stereotype and unquestionably exacerbates all the distortions of perception already discussed in the three papers. The absence of focus on these sources of distortion no doubt reflects gaps in research, which points to an area worthy of future exploration.

6

Assessing the Functional Status of Older Patients: Its Significance for Therapeutic Management

GEORGE L. MADDOX, Ph.D

Introduction

Health is a societal as well as personal concern, and this personal concern has important interpersonal components. An individual's physical and mental capacity to perform in a broad range of social roles obviously has personal significance. Parsons' intuition that most sick persons can be expected to want to feel and be better and to want to seek help to feel and be better is surely borne out by experience and evidence (Parsons, 1975). And, insofar as being ill is assumed in the typical case to be "unmotivated" and not attributed to personal irresponsibility, the sick person can be granted conditional relief from usual role obligations and can expect supportive behavior from kin, friends, and assorted social helpers, the most prestigious of whom is the physician. The helper-patient role set, consequently, has received a great deal of attention; and, not surprisingly, the physician-patient relationship has been of special interest. For purposes of this book on older patients, it is worth noting that Parsons' discussion of the sick role, the essence of which is dependency, has a generational but not a life-cycle emphasis. The physician-patient relationship is an analog of the father-child relationship in his view, without reference to the location of "the child" in the life cycle.

Having been at the periphery of medical sociology for the past few years, in preparation for writing this chapter I reviewed Gallagher's recent volume (1978) whose title, *The Doctor-Patient Relationship in the Changing Health Scene*, promised to bring me up to date. This volume's 455 pages did indeed teach me something. The most important lesson was that, while the health scene may be changing a great deal, our understanding of the doctor-patient relationship has not advanced very much, particularly not in regard to understanding illness behavior over the course of life. For example, the authors of the papers in that volume did not find a single occasion to introduce a life-course perspective in explicating doctor-patient relationships. The index does not reference age or any of its correlates; there is only one reference to an older person, and this appears in an anecdotal illustration. In a society in which there is a national preoccupation with health status of older persons and the high demand and high cost of caring for older persons, this omission is startling. By implication, the age of the patient is not a relevant consideration in understanding doctor-patient relationships.

The dominant motif of Gallagher's volume is professional (specifically, the physician's) dominance and the challenges that are, or in the opinion of the authors, ought to be directed toward modifying that dominance. Parsons' sick role is revisited and appropriately modified by emphasizing the social and societal contexts in which both physicians and patients operate. The "two worlds" of physicians and patients are also revisited; but, while the backgrounds of physicians that affect their behavior when they meet are stressed, surprisingly little empirical evidence about actual encounters is presented.

Three points in Gallagher's volume did get my attention as potentially important for the argument to be developed in this chapter on the health-relevant characteristics of older persons. The first notable point addressed the concept of *role distance* in understanding the behavior of both patients and physicians. An individual may understand a social role, its role set, and its related behavioral expectations, and may even be socially committed to play the role without necessarily being effectively involved in the playing. Although one of Goffman's favorite illustrations of role distancing was the physician maneuvering to remain emotionally in control of the physician-patient role set, physicians might prefer the illustration of the sick patient who expresses role distance through denial of illness. This chapter, however, concentrates on the behavior of physicians who by training and oath are committed to serve patients without regard to color or creed or, one might add, gender or age. In recent years, physicians have gotten a lot of bad press for avoiding nursing homes and for appearing to prefer younger patients. That is, physicians appear to avoid, and to avoid learning about, role sets in which the patient is older. Specifically, I will argue in this chapter that, in regard to avoiding or wanting to avoid older persons, physicians, like laymen, are the products of their culture, perhaps more so. They share the dominant preference for the conspicuous productivity stereotypically associated with younger adults, and they want to rescue individuals from illness. As professional performers who like winning more than losing, physicians prefer to be in the "life business" rather than in the "death business." Physicians have been taught to work with children and adults but not how to work with older adults. And they engage in the same kind of common sense cost-benefit, marginal utility analysis as the rest of us: they prefer to work on or work with individuals who are expected to repay that work with many years of productivity. From this perspective, investing in the relatively young has intuitive appeal to physicians as well as societal resource allocators generally. Insofar as the *old* are perceived to be irrevocably impaired, declining, dying, and beyond help, it is hardly surprising that physicians might be found among those distancing themselves from encounters with older patients. Fortunately, physicians are exposed to countervailing ideological and political pressure to assist as well as they can all patients who present themselves. Physicians, therefore, are conflicted pragmatists who might be expected to respond to information that promises to aid them in assisting patients perceived to be unattractive, difficult, and unrewarding. What kinds of information might assist them? Consider the next point.

The second relevant point for this chapter in the Gallagher volume can be captured in the word *differentiated*. Studies of ethnic and racial prejudice and discrimination have suggested that vigorous discrimination is conditioned not only by the presence or absence of vigorous social control but also by the presence or absence of unambiguous, unchallenged negative stereotypes. Avoidance or minimum commitment to the care of older patients by a physician is a form of discrimination toward the old that reflects minimal professional sanctions against such behavior and relatively unrelieved negative stereotypes both of the health status of the older patients and of the potential benefits of therapeutic intervention for such patients. In short, physicians can themselves be victimized by prevailing negative stereotypes of older patients. Until recently, medical educators have not given explicit attention to the geriatric patient in inpatient, outpatient, and community settings. Daniel Federman, M.D., a Harvard Medical School Internist and Chairman of the Board of Internal Medicine, challenged this neglect forcefully this past year in unpublished testimony before the Institute of Medicine's Committee on Geriatric Education. Dr. Federman asserted that the neglect of geriatrics in medical education approaches irresponsibility, and indicated the Board examinations in internal medicine in the future will require knowledge of geriatric disease and therapeutics. Older patients are not an undifferentiated collectivity about whom nothing is known and for whom nothing effective can be done; we already know more than is implemented in practice. Moreover, he volunteered, the effective teaching of geriatrics will have to be done to a substantial degree outside the confines of the highly centralized, highly technological medical centers. This will be necessary in order to insure that an adequate sampling of older persons as well as older patients can be experienced and that different levels of functioning among older patients can be appreciated. This observation leads to a third point.

A notable focal point in the Gallagher volume is found in a discussion of *client-centered technology*. The centralized medical facility that features inpatient services and high technology is the hallmark of contemporary medical care. This characterization is at least partly accurate, and is the occasion not only for Illich's (1975) complaint about "medicalization" of social life but also of complaints by numerous health care professionals and economists who feel our society institutionalizes too many sick people for too long and subjects them to questionably effective technology at a very high cost. Interest is, therefore, understandably increasing in some client-centered technologies that feature improved patient assessment and triage and also community-based services depending heavily on informal social support networks. This chapter will argue that some "soft" technology such as client assessment can indeed play an important complementary role in the care process. Effective patient care assessment procedures can assist, when a physician and an older patient meet, by helping to break the undifferentiated stereotype of the older patient and by providing a useful point of departure for therapeutic management.

Narrowing the Focus

This chapter concentrates on a specific aspect of encounters between professional helpers and older persons, that is, comprehensive assessment of functional status. Please note the designations *professional helpers* and *older persons*. Professional helper is meant to designate not only physicians but also a broad array of clinicians and program specialists who are responsible for and involved in the care of older persons. Both experience and evidence, in my judgment, make it axiomatic that the well-being of older persons—perhaps of any person, for that matter—cannot be reduced to or effectively achieved by medical care alone. The care process is a complex, differentiated process; understanding how to package the components of that process efficiently and effectively is understandably one of the priority tasks of a society with a predictably aging population. *Older person* refers to a highly differentiated collectivity with various degrees of impairment and various personal and social resources. An accurate characterization of the differentiated collectivity of older persons is socially important as a challenge to prevailing stereotypes. An accurate characterization is also professionally important as a means for anticipating and for responding to the ways in which older patients present themselves to helping professionals.

Ways of thinking about older people—assessment strategies, to use clinical language—have practical consequences. This chapter outlines a way of thinking about older persons that has come to be the shared perspective of a large number of colleagues at the Duke University Center for the Study of Aging and Human Development in recent years. This way of thinking is called the Older American Resources and Services (OARS) strategy (Maddox & Dellinger, 1978). OARS is an information system that is more than a way of thinking about older people and older patients. It is a way of thinking about the care process: intake, diagnosis, treatment planning and implementation, and follow-up in the interest of assessing the effectiveness of intervention. OARS is also a way of thinking about competency-based clinical training and a way of thinking about the effectiveness of programs designed to maintain or increase the well-being of older persons. The first component of the Duke information system is a Multidimensional Functional Assessment Questionnaire (the MFAQ); this procedure is the focus of our attention here.

This chapter then, is intended to illustrate how systematic assessment of functional status can make a contribution to therapeutic management of older persons. The Duke patient assessment procedure is not the only way of characterizing older patients nor the best way for all purposes. In any case, my purpose in this brief presentation is not a comparative evaluation of alternative patient strategies but an illustration of a single strategy and how it has been used with beneficial effect on the behavior of clinicians and on the therapeutic management of older patients.

The OARS Strategy

In 1972 the Duke Center was asked by a federal agency to address what was then called "the alternatives to institutionalization" issue (Maddox, 1972). Congress was distressed by the high and increasing cost of caring for older persons and particularly by assertions, partially confirmed by evidence, that large numbers of older persons were unnecessarily and ineffectively institutionalized. My colleagues and I conceptualized the problem we were asked to address as follows. These colleagues were an assortment of clinicians (physicians, social workers, psychologists), methodologists, system analysts, and economists.

The notion of alternative care strategies called to mind that older persons are the unwitting—and sometimes unwilling—participants in a number of quasi experiments created by legislation that affect the availability and structure of services. Older persons are, therefore, subjected differentially to an existing array of services; this fact presents an opportunity for assessing the efficiency and effectiveness of observed alternatives. For assessing the impact of naturally occurring quasi experiments, patient classification plays a central role. For example, if one can define the essential characteristics of older persons at a Time 1, identify the services to which those persons were exposed over a period of time, and then reassess the status of these persons at a Time 2, one can characterize how various naturally occurring service systems operate. Such information is not routinely collected; getting appropriate information is clearly a very formidable task. We initially directed our attention to a challenging but more manageable task: developing reliable, valid procedures for characterizing older persons and characterizing service systems.

In regard to procedures for functional assessment of older persons and patients, the literature provided an embarrassment of riches (e.g., Duke, 1978, Ch. 2). We found characterizations of older persons that stressed economic status, social resources, mental status, physical status, capacity for self care, or some combination of two of these. Our experienced clinicians were sure that at least these five dimensions ought to be in an equation of well-being, so we constructed the Multidimensional Functional Assessment Questionnaire (MFAQ) designed to produce SEMPA ratings. SEMPA is an acronym for five dimensions of functioning: Social, Economic, Mental, Physical, and Activities of Daily Living (self-care capacity). The derivation and technical aspects of the SEMPA ratings have been described elsewhere (Maddox & Dellinger, 1978); but several general observations about methodology are relevant here. The components of the SEMPA ratings have passed all of the usual tests of reliability and validity; they are quantifiable and are machine scorable; the various SEMPA dimensions are appropriately orthogonal; and they are designed so that the same instrument can be used for clinical intake (i.e., clinicians are comfortable with them for characterizing an individual) and in epidemiological surveys (i.e., social survey analysis are comfortable in generating characterizations of populations). This last characteristic should be stressed because, in the discussion of older persons and patients, clinicians and resource allocators, who typically place very different emphases on individuals and populations, both benefit from the common reference provided by the OARS MFAQ information. One should also note that the MFAQ concentrates on functioning, not on disease or pathological state (see Shanas & Maddox, 1976). A SEMPA rating or profile is intended to be value-free; that is, it can be used to describe well-being and adequate functioning as well as disease or impairment.

The OARS strategy, in addition to a characterization of individual and population well-being, includes a procedure for disaggregating and reaggregating service systems into 25 standardized, generic service components. Since this chapter is about the systematic functional assessment of older patients the service system analysis issue will not be pursued (see Duke, 1978). However, the importance of the disaggregation procedure will surely be intuitively obvious. There is no procedure currently available for characterizing service systems in a standard way. Yet such a characterization is crucial for measuring service system interventions and for conceptualizing alternative interventions. An alternative intervention is, after all, some difference in the packaging of service components in terms of what is offered, by whom, and where.

Characterizing Older Persons and Patients

The OARS MFAQ has been used by a network of over 50 clinicians and research investigators nationwide. I will concentrate here primarily on two large epidemiological studies involving probability samples of 998 persons 65 years of age or older in Durham County, North Carolina, and of 1,609 older persons in Cleveland, Ohio, and secondarily on several smaller studies in North Carolina (see Duke, 1978; Maddox & Dellinger, 1978; Laurie, 1978). What kinds of SEMPA profiles of older persons emerge?

1. In both Durham (59 percent) and Cleveland (57 percent), most older people are *not* functionally impaired on any of the five SEMPA dimensions (Table 6–1). In this case, the 6-point SEMPA ratings are dichotomized and produce 32 categories or profiles of impairment.
2. If older persons in these two communities are functionally impaired, they tend to be multiply impaired (also Table 6–1). One rarely observes an older person who is impaired only in physical functioning or only in mental functioning, for example. But although multiple impairments are common, the category of older persons who might be considered at very high risk of institutionalization (e.g., mental or physical impairment matched with social isolation and poverty) is relatively low (about 2 percent) in both studies.
3. The similarities in functional profiles (Table 6–1) and in the distribution of SEMPA categories in the populations of the two studies are substantial (Table 6–2; SEMPA rating trichotomized). The largest difference observed is in terms of economic well-being, with the Durham black subsample being disadvantaged when compared to their counterparts in Cleveland.

4. Subsamples within older populations have strikingly different SEMPA profiles (Table 6–3). For example, a subsample of persons 75 years of age displays significant elevations in impairment on every dimension and a subsample 80 years of age and older even more so. Blacks tend to be more impaired on every dimension than whites; women tend to be slightly more impaired than men; marital

TABLE 6–1
Patterns of Functional Dimensions
(SEMPA) Durham and Cleveland

| | Percentages | |
SEMPA*	Durham (N = 998)	Cleveland (N = 1609)
OOOOO	58.5	56.7
OOOOX	2.3	2.0
OOOXO	5.6	11.2
OOOXX	5.7	3.7
OOXOO	1.0	1.3
OOXOX	0.6	0.7
OOXXO	1.0	1.2
OOXXX	4.7	3.7
OXOOO	5.1	3.7
OXOOX	0.6	0.1
OXOXO	1.9	1.3
OXOXX	1.1	0.8
OXXOO	0.4	0.3
OXXOX	0.8	0.3
OXXXO	0.5	0.8
OXXXX	1.2	1.1
XOOOO	3.0	4.4
XOOOX	0.2	0.1
XOOXO	0.8	1.4
XOOXX	0.9	0.6
XOXOO	0.3	0.4
XOXXO	—	0.4
XOXOX	0.1	—
XOXXX	1.0	0.1
XXOOO	0.5	1.4
XXOOX	—	0.1
XXOXO	0.1	0.6
XXOXX	0.4	0.2
XXXOO	0.6	0.5
XXXOX	0.3	0.1
XXXXO	0.5	0.4
XXXXX	0.3	0.3

*SEMPA = Social, Economic, Mental Health,
   Physical Health, Activities of Daily Living.
X = Impaired (score of 4–6).
O = Unimpaired (score of 1–3).
Source: Maddox and Dellinger (1978).

TABLE 6–2
Distribution of Functional Status in Two Populations on Five Dimensions

Rating	Social		Economic		Mental Health		Physical Health		Activities of Daily Living	
	Cleveland	Durham	Cleveland	Durham	Cleveland	Durham	Cleveland	Durham	Cleveland	Durham
*Excellent or good	70	73	52	44	68	64	41	43	64	64
†Mildly or moderately impaired	25	24	46	54	28	32	53	47	30	27
‡Severely or completely impaired	5	3	2	2	2	4	4	5	9	10

*Excellent/good is equivalent to 1 or 2 on the uniform 6-point scale.
†Mild or moderate impairment is equivalent to 3 or 4 on the uniform 6-point scale.
‡Severe impairment is equivalent to 5 or 6 on the uniform 6-point scale.
Source: Maddox and Dellinger (1978).

TABLE 6–3
OARS Community Survey, Durham, North Carolina:
Percentage of Population Impaired[a] on Each of the Five Dimensions

| | Total | Age | | | Race | | Sex | | Marital Status | | | |
		65–74 yrs.	75+	80+	White	Black	Male	Female	Married	Widowed	Single Separated Divorced	Total
Social Resources	9	9	8	8	7	14	8	10	4	12	18	9
Economic Resources	14	13	16	16	9	26	11	16	8	20	20	14
Mental Health	13	10	18	22	10	17	14	12	9	14	23	13
Physical Health	25	22	34	44	24	28	26	25	21	29	30	25
ADL	21	14	36	52	19	23	19	22	15	25	27	21
	N=998	N=662	N=315	N=154	N=656	N=341	N=373	N=624	N=440	N=462	N=95	N=998

[a]SEMPA ratings dichotomized.
Source: Duke Center, 1978.

status is associated with functioning with those who are currently married presenting the most favorable profiles.

5. The SEMPA profiles of patients or clients in different service settings are strikingly different (Table 6–4). When clients/patients in a family medicine clinic, a geriatric evaluation and treatment clinic, long-term care institutions, and adult day care in Durham, North Carolina, are compared with the Durham and Cleveland community profiles, expectedly the community samples exhibit a higher level of well-being. The various service settings attract individuals with different SEMPA profiles, that is, institutionalized persons have very high impairment scores. The family service patients have an elevated level of physical impairment and elevated social and economic impairments but a level of mental health impairment no higher than that observed in the community samples. The geriatric evaluation and treatment clinic patients exhibit impairments at a level much higher than the community samples but lower than the institutionalized sample. The exception is mental health, where the clinic sample is more impaired; this exception is explained, at least in part, by the perception of this clinic by professionals as par-

TABLE 6–4
Percentage of Functionally Impaired Clients
Served by North Carolina's Adult Day Care Centers
Compared with Findings of Other Surveyed Populations

Functional Dimension	N.C. Adult Day Care (N = 119)	Durham Co. Institutions (N = 102)	Duke OARS Clinic (N = 98)	Duke-Watts Family Medicine (N = 130)	Durham Community (N = 998)	Cleveland Community (N = 1,609)
Social Resources	17	66	41	32	9	11
Economic Resources	40	49	45	33	14	12
Mental Health	22	71	81	13	13	12
Physical Health	41	60	49	58	25	28
ADL	34	93	60	28	21	14
Cumulative Impairment Scores (CIS)[a]	25	87	50	25	12	9

[a]*CIS is derived as follows: each of the 5 SEMPA dimensions is scored on a 6 point scale with 1 = no impairment and 6 = maximum impairment. Summing the scores for the 5 dimensions produces a range from 5 to 30 with the midpoint 17.5. In this table percent impaired means percent with CIS greater than 17.5.*
Source: Bias and Crawford, 1979.

ticularly appropriate for older persons with mental health problems.

6. Some older persons observed in community samples (we estimate
   about 12 percent) have profiles of impairment at a level usually
   seen primarily among institutionalized older persons (Duke, 1978;
   Laurie, 1978).
7. And, among significantly impaired older persons living in the community, a substantial amount of the care received is provided by informal networks of kin and friends (Laurie, 1978).

In sum, application of the OARS functional assessment procedure reveals a highly differentiated older population. A majority of older individuals appears to be functionally adequate. Those exhibiting impairments re-
veal a variety of patterns; these patterns are differentially distributed in
various service settings.

Some Uses of OARS Profiles

The availability of a reliable, valid, quantifiable, easily used procedure for
multidimensional characterization of older individuals and populations has
led to a number of applications that have potential for affecting therapeutic
management of impaired individuals in beneficial ways.

Population Profiles. As noted in the previous section, epidemiological studies and the accumulation of intake profiles in various service
settings have generated descriptive information that emphasizes variations in functional capacity within older populations and between the
various settings in which they are observed. The dominant observation
is the functional adequacy of the average older person and the difference in functional profiles observed in different settings. The importance of these observations for training health professionals can be illustrated in several ways. Recently, Marc Weksler, Wright Professor
of Geriatric Medicine at Cornell, asserted in a public address at Duke
University, that in the training of physicians, the trainee must have an
opportunity to use the full range of functioning known to exist in older
populations. To observe only the very impaired older patient reinforces
prevalent and misleading stereotypes. This is similar to the comments
of Federman noted earlier. Also, in Duke's mandatory geriatric rotation for residents in family medicine and internal medicine, the importance of seeing the older person in a variety of settings—at home, in
the ambulatory clinic, in the acute hospital, and in long-term care settings—is stressed for the same reason. The differentiated OARS functional profiles provide accessible documentation of patterned variation

in functioning in older persons, which clinicians profitably keep in mind when their work requires concentration on subsamples of that population in various clinical settings (Moore & Kane, 1979).

Planning and Staffing Services. When the Duke Center's Geriatric Evaluation, Treatment and Family Service Clinic was being designed four years ago, the available OARS profile of Durham County's older persons figured importantly in making decisions about services and staffing. The predecessor of the clinic had emphasized geropsychiatric services. The observed configurations of impairments in the OARS survey (Table 6–1) suggested, however, that mental health impairments alone would rarely be presented. This led us to provide in the clinic services and staff not only for psychiatry and social work but also for internal medicine and nursing. Experience has confirmed the wisdom of this decision (Table 6–4); among the impaired, multiple impairments are the rule.

Since the potential of the MFAQ as an intake instrument as well as an epidemiological survey instrument was known, we decided to build the OARS profiles into our basic clinical information system. The initial MFAQ for each patient seen in the center's clinic is recorded in an on-line computer system, and is available for staffing conferences where decisions are made regarding the need for additional information and where diagnosis and patient management plans are made. Additional information from the staffing conferences also becomes part of the on-line clinical record.

As cases have accumulated, it has become possible for a senior or student clinician to ask and answer the following kinds of questions. When a patient is seen for the first time, the clinician can ask, "Have we seen a profile like this before? How often? For patients with a given type of profile, what kinds of special tests or additional information have usually been requested? What are the most common diagnoses? What are the typical management plans?" Since, as a matter of policy, clinic patients are followed up at least at six-month intervals, as cases accumulate it will be possible to inquire about the relationships among management plans, their implementation, the cost of implementation, and their consequences. We call this information system "The Living Textbook of Geriatric Care." It is a variant of the Duke Department of Medicine's well-known "Living Textbook of Cardiology" (Rosati et al., 1975).

Clinical Training. The Living Textbook of Geriatric Care is intended to stress the multidimensional aspects of a continuous care process. There are many indications it succeeds with clinical trainees. Students from a wide variety of professional backgrounds (the Center's clinic trains about 70 professionals annually) are exposed to a common frame of reference for characterizing the functional status of older persons, and learn how to translate this characterization in relevant ways to the diagnostic, management planning, and assessment of effectiveness phases of the care processes.

In family medicine, the OARS functional assessment strategy has been used in an instructive clinical experiment not yet published. Using an experimental, switch-over controlled comparison, Moore provided experimental subjects (family physicians) SEMPA profiles of their older ambulatory patients at the time of the first contact, and then audited patient records (Family Medicine at Duke uses the Weed Problem Oriented Record) to determine whether the information on functioning affected the problems noted and the problems managed. For comparison, he audited the patient records of residents who were not supplied this information.The outcome was not exactly what Moore anticipated. The impact of the SEMPA information did not make a significant difference in the entries found in case records. However, the family physicians exposed to the SEMPA information requested additional training in the comprehensive diagnosis and care of older patients. In fact, this experiment initiated a series of training activities that resulted in an innovative and flourishing geriatric focus within the family program, which features multidimensional functional assessment and training experience in ambulatory clinic, hospital, long-term care, community, and home settings.

As noted earlier, part of the OARS assessment strategy, in addition to the SEMPA ratings, generates information about the services impaired individuals report receiving and from whom. This information plus additional information gathered directly from service agencies (Laurie, 1978) makes it very clear that most of the services received by older persons are provided by kin and friends. This is extremely relevant information for clinicians as well as for service planners and resource allocators (Bias & Crawford, 1979). The availability of informal social support can make the difference between institutionalization and remaining in the community.

Conclusions

In a social context said to be characterized by negative, undifferentiated older persons, clinicians can benefit from the person-centered technology represented by the OARS multidimensional functional assessment and its related procedure for service system characterization. This is so not because the OARS stategy is demonstrably the only way to think about functioning in later life (it is not) or is the best way to think about functioning (there is no best way). OARS is a useful tool that demonstrably crosses disciplinary boundaries with some ease, illustrates the complexity of the average older person in understandable terms, can be related to the total care process, and can be integrated into an information system in which the effectiveness of our interventions can be tested.

I call OARS a useful tool with the following story in mind. Twenty years ago, when I arrived at Duke, Morton Bogdonoff was professor of medicine and chief of the outpatient clinic. At morning report at 7 A.M., he would frequently say, "Doctors, pay attention. What I am about to tell you will make you get up tomorrow morning with greater enthusiasm for your work, and will help you end the day with great satisfaction." This is what I have come to feel about the OARS strategy. It works in ways that provide a realistic basis for optimism about the functional capacity of older people and about our capacity to understand and deal with their incapacity in therapeutically useful ways when intervention is necessary. An accurate information system is not equivalent to effective therapeutic intervention. But it is a first and important step. An accurate information system that can be used to identify useful interventions does not provide a simple answer to societal negativism regarding later life. But appropriate differentiation of the functional capacity of older persons is a first and important step.

7
Experiencing Symptoms: Attribution and Misattribution of Illness among the Aged

CARY KART, Ph.D.

This chapter deals with the illness behavior of older people. In particular, I am interested in how aged people experience symptoms and what influences how they come to decide they are ill. A context for this discussion is established by outlining some problems basic to defining health and illness and by briefly introducing the notion of the illness career.

Defining Health and Illness

A broad consensus appears to exist in this society about the desirability of good health. Interestingly, however, although it seems to be taken for granted that everyone knows what "health" means, few attempts have been made to define the term substantively. A notable exception to this is the definition of health put forth by the World Health Organization (WHO) in the late 1940s, although the argument has been made that this definition (". . . a state of complete physical, mental, and social well-being and not merely the absence of disease or infirmity") is so all-encompassing as to make matters only worse (Callahan, 1977). Some argue that it may be more useful to attempt to define illness. As Callahan points out, most people in most places have a rough idea of what is meant by "ill"; and, even if the borderlines are fuzzy, a recognizable area of human experience is evoked by the term.

Unfortunately, many are *too* familiar with this area of human experience. It is probably rare that individuals find themselves in a continuous state of being free of bodily stimuli that are capable of being interpreted as illness symptoms. Robinson (1971) notes that it is not uncommon in health surveys to discover that upwards of 90 percent of apparently healthy subjects report the presence of clinical symptoms or disorders worthy of treatment. Most of these "illnesses" are never brought to the attention of health care professionals (Kosa & Robertson, 1969). Complicating matters is that when they are brought to professionals, there is often disagreement about diagnosis. In addition, it may be useful to point out that although the leading cause of morbidity and mortality in the United States once was acute infectious disease, today chronic diseases have taken on increasing importance. Many diabetics, hypertensives, survivors of heart attacks, and others do not usually feel sick; they may function effectively in jobs and their other social roles. Should they be regarded as ill or healthy?

All societies must manage the problem of defining health and illness. This is so because a society's survival is based on ensuring that members of the population can perform certain fundamental tasks. Thus, health can be seen as a functional requisite of societies, and as Parsons (1958, 1965) points out, "there must . . . always be standards of adequacy of . . . performance and . . . a corresponding set of distinctions between states of individuals which are and are not satisfactory from the point of view of these standards." From this perspective, health (and illness) may be defined with references to the social roles and performance tasks the individual carries out in the society, rather than in biological terms.

This normative approach is certainly not without problems. One involves the extent to which nonphysiological states may influence the determination of health or illness. Rosenstock and Kirscht (1979) offer the example of two men who have had recent myocardial infarctions. One is a white-collar worker who is able to return to his job; the other is a blue-collar worker who will have to change jobs in order to return to work. From a normative position, the former would be regarded as healthy and the latter ill. In addition, if "standards of performance" are age biased, then it is possible from a normative point of view to define a large proportion of all aged individuals as ill.

One way out of the definitional problem of health and illness may be to concentrate on health-related and illness-related behavior. Health behavior involves the health-maintenance activity undertaken by a person who believes himself or herself to be healthy (Kasl & Cobb, 1966). Illness behavior refers to the ways in which given symptoms may be differentially perceived, evaluated, and acted (or not acted) upon by individuals (Mechanic, 1961). The notion of sick role behavior is included under the definition of illness behavior. Baric (1969) has suggested the concept of the "at risk" role to describe individuals who are somewhere between the state of health and the state of experiencing symptoms of illness. Such individuals are at higher risk to illness than the population at large.

The Illness Career

Julius Roth (1963:93) has written that "when people go through the same series of events, we speak of this as a career and of the sequence and tim- of events as their career timetable." Roth used the institutionalized TB patient as his career model. He argued that individuals involved in an ill- ness career try to define when certain salient illness-related events will happen to them. Individuals develop time norms against which to measure their individual progress. The benchmarks on this timetable are the signi- ficant events that occur in the average career. Roth depicts the TB patient as attempting to "speed up" his illness career in order to move as quickly as possible toward the goal of restored health.

Gustafson (1972) has applied Roth's notion of career timetables to the home setting. She views the last phase of life as a career that moves in a series of related stages toward death. These stages, she argues, are defined by a series of "benchmarks," which, for the elderly patients, con- sist of the degree of deterioration indicated by their social activity, mobili- ty, and physical and mental functioning. A "successful" career in this sense consists of the slowest possible regression from one stage to another. However, for most people, old and young alike, unlike Gustafson's nursing home patients, a "successful" illness career consists of the fastest possible movement from illness to health.

Each episode of illness can also be viewed in a career sense. Several early attempts were made to define stages of the illness career. For the most part, these schemata emphasized psychological factors as influencers of the way people define and experience their illness career. For example, Barker and his associates (1946) distinguished between stages of illness and convalescence. During the illness stage, people suffer confinement and reduced mobility. In addition, the sick person's concern about the outcome of the illness tends to limit attention to matters of physical condition. These behaviors have a way of reinforcing a preoccupation with self to the exclusion of other interests. The convalescence stage is characterized by a renewal of strength and interests in the outside world. Lederer (1958) added the stage of "becoming sick" to Barker's schema. This stage in- volves the period of experiencing symptoms, the anxiety associated with them, and all that is involved in coming to define oneself as ill.

A more recent formulation by Suchman (1965) separates the illness experience into five stages and describes them in terms of social, cultural, and psychological factors. The stages include:

1. symptom experience,
2. assumption of the sick role,

3. medical care contact,
4. dependent-patient role, and
5. recovery or rehabilitation.

This conceptual schema is an ideal type and attempts to describe a typical behavior sequence. Obviously, these stages need not manifest themselves in the behavior of every individual. Below, I confine myself to the beginning stage of the illness career, the symptom experience stage, and discuss factors affecting the attribution and misattribution of illness among the aged.

The Physical Experience of Symptoms

It is in the symptom experience stage that the illness career begins, for it is here that the individual first may begin to perceive that something is wrong. There are two analytically distinguishable aspects of the symptom experience:

1. the physical experience, by which is meant the pain, discomfort, or awareness of a change in appearance or functioning, and
2. the cognitive aspect, which involves the evaluation and interpretation of the physical experience.

Emotional response may accompany the physical experience and/or the cognitive evaluation.

Suchman (1965) selected 137 cases involving disturbing illness symptoms from his larger survey of 5,340 persons residing in a community of New York City. This subsample, two-thirds of whom were 45 years of age or older, included adults who, during the two months prior to the interview, either required three or more physician visits and were incapacitated for five or more consecutive days or required hospitalization for one or more days. Suchman found that pain was by far the most important initial warning sign that something was wrong; it was mentioned by 66 percent of the respondents. Fever or chills or shortness of breath were less important initial symptoms and were expressed by 17 percent and 10 percent of the respondents, respectively. In a majority or near-majority of cases, respondents reported that the symptoms were severe, continuous, incapacitating and unalleviated. In general, these data are consistent with a body of literature that supports the notion that more visible symptoms are more readily experienced and defined.

As Rodin (1978) points out, feedback from physiological processes is not usually monitored at the conscious level when everything is working

smoothly. Yet, even when things are not working smoothly (physiological-
ly speaking), an individual's recognition and tolerance for physiological responses such as pain may vary as a function of social and/or cultural variables. For example, Zborowski (1952) studied ethnic reactions to pain in a
VA hospital, and observed that Jewish and Italian patients responded to
pain in an emotional fashion, but "old Americans" were more stoical, and
Irish patients frequently denied pain. Further, attitudinal differences
were noted to underlie the Italian and Jewish concern with pain. Zborowski reports that although the Italian patients primarily sought relief from
pain, the Jewish patients were mainly concerned with the meaning and
significance of their pain and the consequences of pain for their future welfare and health. Zborowski attributes these different responses to pain to
cultural differences in familial response to the health and illness of the patients when they were children. Additional studies inside the laboratory
(Sternback & Tursky, 1965) and outside of it (Zola, 1966) support Zborowski's findings.

Age itself may also have an impact on the recognition of physiological
responses such as pain and elevated temperature. In the elderly, pain normally associated with a disease process may not be present. This is because the traditional clinical picture associated with a disease often under-
goes age-related changes. The chest pain associated with angina pectoris is
sometimes absent. Pathy (1967) noted that one-fifth of elderly patients
who suffered heart attacks exhibited no pain. Likewise, the abdominal
pain that normally accompanies an appendicitis attack may not be present
in an older victim. An elevated temperature that normally accompanies
various diseases, especially acute infectious episodes, may be absent or
late in appearing in the older individual. In addition, because of reduced
sensitivity, elderly individuals may not respond to the elevated tempera-
tures that accompany infections. This evidence suggests that the illnesses
of elderly individuals may be further along than those of younger persons
at the time of physical recognition of symptoms.

Evaluation of Symptoms

People experiencing changes in usual body functioning try to make sense
of their experiences. This often takes the form of hypotheses regarding the
possible cause of symptoms. A central issue in most perceptions of causality is whether to attribute a given experience to internal or external states
(Freedman, Sears, & Carlsmith, 1978). External attribution would ascribe
causality to anything external to the individual, such as the general environment, role constraints or role losses, stressful tasks he or she may be

working on, and so on. Internal causes include such factors as disease states, biological aging, personality, or mood and motivation (Freedman, Sears, & Carlsmith, 1978).

Potentially, the development of illness attribution and misattribution can be affected by many factors internal and external to the individual. Among these are included the perceived seriousness of symptoms, the extent of disruption of normal activities involved, the frequency and persistence of the symptoms, the amount of pain and discomfort to which a person is used, the medical knowledge of the person, the need to deny illness, the nature of competing needs, the availability of alternative explanations, and the accessibility of treatment (Mechanic, 1978). Sex (Nathanson, 1975), social class (Koos, 1954; Andersen, Anderson, & Smedby, 1968; Osborn, 1973), and the presence of a lay referral system (Friedson, 1960, 1961) also affect how symptoms are evaluated and defined.

According to Jones and Nisbett (1971), actors and observers tend to make different causal attributions. Actors usually see their behavior as a response to an external situation in which they find themselves, but, typically, observers attribute the same response to factors internal to the actor. This difference between an actor's and an observer's attributions can be expected to lead to misunderstanding and, perhaps, especially so in a health-care context. Patients and their physicians may see the same event from different perspectives. The patient attributes his response to environmental factors (e.g., stress at home) that are out of the purview of the physician, but the physician attributes the patient's response to internal physical processes (e.g., disease states, biological aging). These internal processes are, for the most part, the only causal explanations available to the physician; he may be handicapped by a lack of information about what the actor may be responding to in his environment.

This is the stuff of which problems in the doctor-patient relationship are made. The noncompliant patient may be deemed uncooperative or recalcitrant by the physician ("the patient has a personality problem"); the patient attributes his noncompliance to situational factors (e.g., the medication made him sick, he was not given enough information, support, or motivation by the physician) (Janis & Rodin, 1979).

Interestingly, the elderly themselves seem overly ready to make attributions to internal physical processes rather than to the environment (Janis & Rodin, 1979). Their perceptions often include grossly exaggerated notions of what happens during normal aging. Too many associate pain and discomfort, debilitation or decline in intellectual function with aging per se. These are not normal accompaniments of aging. Unfortunately, such associations are supported by significant others ("What do you expect at your age?") as well as by physicians. In fact, the aged patient-doctor relationship may be a special case of actor-observer interaction when both agree that events are attributable to internal physical processes (e.g., biological aging). This consensus may act to reinforce a set of consequences that are essentially negative. First, elderly individuals may assume that aging has had a greater impact on them than it really has. For example, Kahn and his associates (1975) found that only a small amount of memory loss was evident in an elderly sample, yet a high degree of loss was perceived by patients. These perceptions were highly correlated with depression. Second, they attribute all negative changes in health and mood to aging per se. Chest pain as a warning signal of heart disease may be considered another attack of heartburn; bone pain, which may herald a fracture or bone cancer, may be ascribed to age-related rheumatism. A change in bowel habits is a well-known danger signal of cancer. Such an alteration may easily be ignored by an older person who seems to be plagued by bowel problems. Even rectal bleeding may be attributed by the patient to hemorrhoids.

Elderly persons are more likely than younger persons to develop mental manifestations of their physical problems. Too often, these mental manifestations—mental confusion, and so-called senility—are considered normal accompaniments of aging. Libow (1973) argues that the diagnosis of senility, or what some more accurately refer to as quasi-senility or pseudo-senility, frequently involves misdiagnosis, which can be caused by medications, metabolic imbalance, malnutrition, diminished cardiac output, fever, and respiratory conditions. When these conditions are treated, the "senility" often goes away.

Schouten (1975) reports on the experiences of two elderly individuals in his geriatrics department who were judged mentally confused. On the basis of their perceived mental state, they were to be transferred to a psychogeriatric unit. However, it was found that both of these patients had suffered from heart attacks and that the decreased blood flow to the brain associated with these episodes had been the cause of the confusion. As they recovered from the heart attacks, their mental confusion disappeared. When diseases or physical states result in temporary disorientation in the young, they are often said to be delirious. When such states occur in the elderly, they are said to be mentally confused or senile, and are expected to remain so.

Attributing illness to biological factors may incorrectly focus an elderly person (and his physician) away from situational and social factors that are stress-inducing and affect health. Much gerontological literature is concerned with the impact on health status of retirement, widowhood, and changing living environments, among other factors.

In general, no social science support has been found for the notion that retirement is detrimental to health. Yet, as Butler and Lewis (1973) point out, reconciling social science and clinical data may be difficult because individuals get lost in the mass of data. Butler (1975) has used the term "retirement syndrome" to describe the fact that retirement may be pathogenic to some individuals. Ellison (1968) suggests that some retirees may become "ill" because they define illness as a more legitimate role than being retired. Simon & Cahan (1963) reported that patients with reversible (acute) brain syndromes were likely to have fewer family ties, and their retirement tended to occur before age 65.

It is well established that the mortality rate for many causes of death is much higher among widows and widowers than among married persons of the same age (Parkes, 1964). Kraus and Lilienfeld (1959) showed that the effects of widowhood (grief and accompanying environmental changes) are the most likely causes of this increased mortality. Informative studies having to do with widowhood and morbidity are scarce. One noteworthy report published 35 years ago indicated that the physical reactions to grief experienced by older people included stomach distress, shortness of breath, lack of strength, and "subjective distress" (Lindemann, 1944). Several more recent studies also show increases in physician visits during the first year of bereavement, especially for psychological symptoms (Clayton, 1973).

The relationship of environmental change to mortality and morbidity has been investigated in mental hospitals, nursing homes, and homes for the aged. Moving the older person from a familiar setting into an institution, or even into surroundings similar to his or her own home, has been reported to cause psychological disorganization. Verwoerdt (1976) offers the case of a 74-year-old recluse who lived in an old shack in filth and constant danger of being burned (he used a wood stove to prepare his meals). The old man was persuaded, after great effort, to move into a modern facility with plumbing and electricity. A few days after the move, the social worker received an urgent call about the man. Upon her arrival, she found the man in a state of acute confusion; he was lying in his bed, with evidence of fecal incontinence all around him. Neither disorientation nor fecal incontinence had been a problem before then. Although some researchers might emphasize the stress of relocation involved in the above anecdote, others might focus on environmental discontinuity or the degree of change between a new and old environment. Lawton (1974) believes the newly institutionalized elderly are in double jeopardy in this regard. He argues that individuals with health-related incapacities are less capable than the healthy in adapting to new environmental situations.

Clearly, when individuals exaggerate the effects of normal aging and attribute all negative changes to inevitable aging processes, actions that could be beneficial are not undertaken. This is the case whether the misattribution ignores real disease processes or environmental factors. Sometimes misattribution can have tragic consequences. Unfortunately, reeducating aged individuals about the effects of normal aging may not be effective in correcting incorrect attributions. Preliminary data from studies by Ross, Lepper, and Hubbard (1975) show incorrect attributions tend to persevere. Although this research was not carried out in a health context, it suggests the importance of early education about the effects of normal aging. This may be the only effective device for reducing illness misattribution to aging among the aged.

Summary

The line between health and illness is not objectively defined. Popularly employed definitions of these terms that rely on self-report or a functionalist perspective clearly have problems. A resultant strategy is to fall back on descriptions of health and illness-related behavior.

Suchman (1965) describes illness behavior in terms of a career perspective. This chapter discusses the first stage of the illness career, the symptom experience stage, and what factors affect the attribution and misattribution of illness among the aged.

In general, the elderly make too many attributions to the aging process per se. One reason for this is that they assume that aging has had a greater impact on them than it really has. Overattribution of symptoms to the aging process directs the attention of the elderly person away from real disease and/or environmental factors that may affect health. Such misattributions may have tragic consequences.

8
Problems in the Care of the Aged

HERBERT J. WEISS, M.D.

What I propose to do is to develop further some of the ideas and precepts that have been presented in earlier chapters and to do so by way of clinical examples, or case presentations. The cases in point, by the very nature of this chapter, must be limited only to clinical illustrations; they cannot be cases fully developed in depth. The main purpose of the examples is to allow us to explore some of the sources of the problems that are encountered in the doctor-patient relationship.

Examples of Misdiagnosis

Let me begin with a vignette to illustrate what I have in mind. First, I was asked by a social worker at a nursing home to see an elderly woman in that nursing home. The woman had been going downhill, had been a resident there for a few years, had become progressively more confused and disorganized, and, accordingly, had been transferred to another part of the nursing home better designed to respond to her failing capabilities. Shortly after the move—within a day or two—the patient had a series of falls, one of which resulted in multiple bruises around the face. The social worker asked that I see her, and I did. The physician in charge of the particular service had *not* asked for psychiatric consultation, and there was no reason why he should; nevertheless, I went to see the patient, and I reviewed the chart. I found that she had had difficulties with walking ever since entering the nursing home about three years before, that she used a cane, that she was being seen by the podiatrist, that she was known to have troubles with her feet (for which she wore specially made shoes). She was not receiving any psychotropic medications, she had no neurological disease that would cause incoordination or motor dysfunction. She was clearly demented, and although this condition had progressed, she was not out of control. She did not appear to be particularly depressed, and conversations with her were rather adequate. The physician had commented on her falls, had encouraged nursing staff to keep a closer watch on her. No one had yet thought it best to restrain her in some physical way. He commented that the patient was being seen in podiatry clinic. Podiatry records told nothing about the condition of the patient's feet: I learned this from the nurse and by looking myself. The podiatrist had been content to treat some skin condition with an antibiotic. Now what is the psychiatrist doing with such a problem? I asked to watch the patient walk. She did indeed carry a cane; it was a cane that one would buy perhaps in a drugstore, although it did have a rubber tip. It was clearly too short for her. She held it in her right hand, not well; as she walked her left leg or knee collapsed, and she tended to teeter to the right. But since she carried the cane in her right hand, she braced herself on some of these occasions. However, when I asked her to turn around and walk some more, she shifted the cane to the left hand, the knee buckled, she fell to the right, and I caught her before she injured herself. I gave her a walking frame, and she ambulated much better. At this point, I concluded my consultation, content to recommend that the patient be evaluated in physical therapy by the orthopedist for proper fitting of a cane or for the use of a walker, and with a request that she wear shoes designed for her, not the ones she was wearing.

Now what is the purpose of this clinical illustration? My question is directed to the internist, who is perfectly capable of doing what I did, and does it all the time; why did he not proceed in exactly the same fashion? He read my note, he agreed, and these recommendations were carried out. More importantly, since this falling was going on even before she was moved to this unit, why was the change not made before? I suggest that the reason the patient was brought to this particular unit was because of her progressive dementia; the fact that the patient now needed to be in a much more protected setting obscured any other considerations at this time. The thinking therefore was: she is getting more confused, more and more disorganized, she is bound to be upset at being here, you will have to watch her closely. In that way, the preoccupation with the mental impairment momentarily obscured the need for a good, solid, physical evaluation. Why did the social worker ask for consultation? I reconstruct his reasoning something like this: the patient was being transferred from a familiar setting. She is reasonably intact and can recognize the changes, she is upset about the changes, perhaps resentful, and now she has symptoms of anxiety, depression, anger, and she responds by falling. He therefore asked for psychiatric consultation so that he might help her make the transfer more readily. It is possible that there is some semblance of truth in this. Yet I contend that the preoccupation with the psychosocial element in the situation obscured the need or the recognition that physical events often have physical origins. The foregoing illustration is an example of a first category of problems that I propose to describe, namely, those arising from missed or incomplete diagnosis and assessment.

A woman in her late seventies has been a patient of the rehabilitation service of a general hospital for more than five weeks. She was admitted on an orthopedic service for removal of the prosthesis previously placed for a fractured hip some time before. The hip was nailed. There was a dislocation with the prosthesis, a second procedure was needed, and now the prosthesis was being removed. Prior to this admission she had functioned pretty well in her own home. She had children who looked in on her; she was quite ambulatory and really quite sharp, intact, and her familiar self. In the hospital, she had failed to respond to any of the physical therapy prescribed for her, absolutely refused to cooperate with it, seemed totally unable to follow any instructions. She complained constantly of pain, or weakness, and for weeks had remained in bed, rarely leaving the room.

The basis for the consultation was more administrative than clinical, although there was plenty of clinical basis for a consultation. Namely, she was exceeding her allotted stay—in fact had exceeded it according to Medicare regulations—and the hospital utilization committee was clamoring for her discharge. The family was resistant because the patient clearly was not performing at an adequate functional level and surely should not have been discharged in that condition. Psychiatric consultation was asked for almost by default. Nursing notes described the patient as frequently confused, disoriented, the word paranoid was regularly encountered, but there was no way of knowing what she had been like before her hospitalization, as no evaluation of the mental status or adequate history of her functioning had really been obtained. It is true that the patient was receiving moderate amounts of tranquilizers of two or three kinds as well as an antidepressant; it was conceivable that one of these drugs in particular might very well have accounted for her current mental status, which seemed to be somewhat lethargic, somewhat confused, and disoriented. She seemed to have a distinct memory deficit, totally unaware of the surgery for which she had entered the hospital, or of any beforehand, and appeared to be quite convincingly demented. I stopped the medication and observed for a week, and there was no change. She continued to be quite clearly demented, except for one early observation. That was the unmistakable expression of recognition when I first came into the room. You see, I had known this patient more than fifteen years before, had treated her for a severe depression, from which she recovered. She knew me instantly, she knew why I was there. None of this appeared to be consonant with the picture of dementia.

The patient was transferred to the psychiatric division, no medications were given, she was urged and encouraged and cajoled into more and more mobilization. She could walk with a walker. She did have distinct shortening of the fractured limb and gait was affected, but she could walk when she chose. She was no longer isolated in her room, but clearly a part, in her way, of the patient community on the unit. Yet in no way did this patient truly respond to the level of independent function of which she was capable, and the motives for this behavior were not difficult to ascertain. She had for many years lived in the same house with one of her daughters, who was chronically and recurrently depressed, and whose character disorder perfectly suited and complemented the mother's character. The daughter, at the time the mother went into the hospital, chose to go away for a short period, and when she returned, and it was time for the mother to go home, she became ill and was readmitted to another psychiatric service. The relationship between mother and daughter living in the same house, in separate suites, was clearly the source of the problem. The patient was not going to get better, the caretaking person was not going to get better, and it was a standoff for the clinician. This part of the case is not particularly important for my consideration; what is significant is the readiness again to ascribe and respond to the patient in terms of the dementia, or to the dementia produced by drugs.

Diagnosis of Dementia

Dementia is clinically described as a disorder that is manifested by impairment of orientation, memory, intellectual function, and judgment, accompanied by lability or perhaps shallowness of the affective range. This pentad of symptoms is indeed classic for moderately advanced dementias, but they may be far from evident when the disorder is mild and in its early stages. And thus such symptoms may be overlooked precisely at a time when treatment might be most effective. There is, on the other hand, considerable evidence that dementia is overdiagnosed, as in the preceding case illustration; that is, that functional disorders are misdiagnosed as organic—particularly, of course, in the aged. There are a number of studies to show this point.

In one study of psychiatric diagnosis given to patients over 65 in three different cities—Toronto, London, and New York—the authors found that organic brain disorders were diagnosed with more than 50 percent greater frequency in New York than in either Toronto or London (Duckworth et al., 1976). Though variations in population may account for some of the difference noted, it seems much more likely that the figures indicate that in New York, elderly patients with affective disorders were labeled as demented, whereas in Great Britain, where many workers have emphasized the importance of recognizing functional disorders in the aged, patients with affective disorder were more likely to be labeled correctly.

Errors of omission and commission in the diagnosis of dementia arise from multiple sources. Failure to recognize the disease when it is present even to a significant degree occurs most commonly simply because the examining physician fails to ask the significant questions. There is a familiar axiom: that physicians have a great tendency to assume answers. I would add to this point that I think other professionals do also. Doctors are not alone. Patients with dementia seldom complain of its characteristic symptoms. Certainly, early in the course of the disease, patients are most likely to complain of somatic discomforts that point perhaps to other diagnoses. We are all familiar with the fact that patients with moderately advanced disease might conceal the dysfunction quite skillfully by using the well-preserved social skills available to them. Diagnosing dementia when it is not present tends to arise from other sources. If the patient appears to be distinctly demented and is not, then the questions asked tend to be appropriate for investigating the possibility of organic brain disease, and usually the examiners get the answer consistent with such a diagnosis. This is exactly the case of the patient I cited. I, too, asked the familiar questions and got the same answers the nursing staff and other physicians in the house were getting. I suppose one might say that this woman was clever enough to know how to answer.

It is necessary to pay close attention to the patient's behavior, not always to the answers to the standard questions. Usually, behavior suggests a level of function compatible with the severity of dysfunction revealed by the mental status examination. When I came in to see the patient, not only did she quickly recognize me and quickly realize why I was there, but she was instantly reabsorbed into the television program she was intently following. There were newspapers on the bedside table, as well as a book, and somehow all this does not add up to being demented. I think another important source of error in diagnosing dementia may stem from our current preoccupation with a new technology, especially with unwarranted reliance on ancillary diagnostic procedures. Here I am speaking of computerized axial tomography, the CAT scan. This patient had had one, too, and she showed the usual degree of cortical atrophy, which may or may not accompany dementia. When the scan is clearly evidential for marked atrophy, the clinical evaluation rarely requires it. In borderline situations, the scan is hardly to be considered pivotal in making the differential diagnosis. One might say the same thing about psychometric studies, although the distortions or disturbances in the protocols for distinctly organic patients frequently coincide with those which are observed clinically. I do not think that in the early or equivocal states they accurately portray the functional and adaptive capacity of the patient, and surely they give very little information as to the sources of the dysfunction, which are likely to emanate more from psychosocial pressures than from strictly organic ones.

Stereotypes about Aging

The foregoing illustrations were chosen only to illustrate a fairly straightforward point, namely, that the familiar stereotype about aging, that it equals physical or organic deterioration, very frequently clogs our perceptions of the nature of the problem, and the cases become problem cases precisely because of the clogged or distorted perception. At the same time, I wish to call attention to the existence of other stereotypes, particularly those in the psychological and social science fields. In our pursuit of a truly gerontological viewpoint about aging, the humanistic psychosocial emphasis based on the totality of the person may at times cloud our vision about another familiar axiom about old age: that the capacity to reestablish the automatic, physiologic, regulating mechanism of the human body does indeed progressively fail as the years proceed. It is true that old people get confused, and it is true that old people get upset, and they do get pushed around, and they sometimes fall down because they have bad feet and weak knees, not only because they are helpless and dependent and frightened. Of course, if you have bad feet and are very frightened, you may fall down even more. It is essential to recognize that one cannot separate the diminished capacity for physical adaptation from the older person's need to adapt psychologically to his or her impaired physical functioning, or, for that matter, to impaired social resources.

This observation puts me in mind of a recent, and in my mind, a very commendable educational program in medical gerontology currently underway in a large university hospital. One educational technique was to teach medical students according to an empathic model, that is by way of a technique of teaching the impact of age-related sensory changes. How does it feel to really be an old person, not being able to see well, or to hear well, or to lose your sense of touch? So the students wore eyeglasses with distorting lenses, ear plugs to reduce auditory acuity, their fingertips were coated in order to impair tactile function; they modeled what it is to be old and infirm. Of course, the point of this technique was to overcome the barrier of familiar attitudes toward the aged by trying to show just how it is to be old. In a sense it is a rather naïve exercise because each one of the students who wore those lenses and coated his fingers had a perfectly intact image of himself that protected him from the real feeling. It would be like trying to teach people how to feel for the dying patient when you don't have any real model of what it is to be dying yourself by way of preparation. You can't really feel it because of the narcissistic protective defenses we all enjoy.

All this leads to the ultimate problem with the aged and to the ultimate stereotype: the physicians, and very often the psychiatrist or the social worker or the counselor, find themselves responding more and more mechanically to the older person's complaint with those familiar words, "You will have to learn how to live with it." You will have to learn how to live with your disabling arthritis, with your failing memory, with inflation on a fixed social security income, with the losses of your friends, with the growing disinterest or dislocation from your children. "You will have to learn how to live with it."

Problems of Dependency

A second category of problems encountered with the aged has to do with the patient-physician relationship: those problems that arise from the unreasonable or exaggerated expectation of the patient coupled with those arising from the unreasonable and exaggerated expectations of the doctor. We might label these problems as those arising from the dependency of the aged patient on the physician. Physicians may be inclined to make errors of several kinds in their response to the psychological or emotional needs of the aged. They may encourage the aged patient to live with disability and accept limitations, stating or implying that such things are normal for getting old, that these disabilities are to be expected, that they are inevitable, and that the old person ought to be able to tolerate them. As a consequence, much that is truly remediable in the aged may be neglected because of the comfort of this stereotype, that it is all part of getting old.

It should be evident to us that in the aged the actual physical impairment, and perhaps even the psychological impairment, is likely to be much less disabling than the functional disability. Perhaps it is because the patient is ignorant of what alternatives or options there are for him, or because there is no opportunity to learn how to use or obtain aids to improve function. More important, I think, it is the patients who need to exaggerate and exploit or to provoke exacerbations of their disability, often in a masked way. They may withhold information from the physician, becoming excessively guarded out of fear of the consequences of the revelations. This attitude has its repercussions in the physician's attitude of telling the patient to "learn to live with it." That statement, however, really connotes in the mind of the patient a different message, namely that the physician is saying "Leave me alone, and don't bother me with your demands." For the patient, this sense of abandonment from the very person from whom he or she might expect the most help, tends to aggravate the disability even more.

I call attention to the warnings we frequently receive not to become too sympathetic and too giving to a patient, and I think this is another major error. The older person is fended off because the physician feels that too much sympathy may encourage or provoke unwarranted dependency upon him. What the physician usually verbalizes is that the dependent patient will not function because he will use the relationship as a crutch, leaning too much on the physician. What this attitude fails to take into account is that frequently, within the structure of this dependent support, the patient will become much more self-sufficient: in the absence of that support, whether it be withheld out of fear or anger, the patient will use, exploit, and cling to illness and disability. I suggest that a hopeful recovery might emerge out of the dependency. Physicians have a great deal of trouble recognizing that aged patients are almost universally emotionally dependent and intent on a search for aid from the doctor, and that the nature of the aid they seek far transcends the strictly clinical efforts of the physician in the technical sense alone. It would be both better and easier for us as physicians or as therapists if we recognized the dependency as part of the patient's way of life and utilized that relationship to mobilize the patient's remaining resources within the context of the reassuring supportive relationship.

Physician Frustration with the Aged Patient

Not long ago I had occasion to discuss with a physician his care of a particular patient known to me because I had treated this man more than fifteen years before for a depression. During the past several years this man, now approaching 80, had been under the care of the original internist. He had little or nothing in the way of physical disability, but he was an extremely obsessive and compulsive patient who still continued to work, but was extremely hypochondriacal. The medications he had received over the past several years had included occasional very mild tranquilizers and antidepressants. Usually he came for treatment with low-grade anxiety, and the physician told me that each visit had become an agony for him. The patient came, sat down with a written list of things he wished to discuss. The list was always the same: the careful cataloguing of his general feelings, constantly repeated, a recital of what was going on in his life, what was happening to his wife, to his children, what his worries were, and not much more. I said to the physician, "What is the problem? He seems to be doing quite well, and you are obviously doing quite well with him; why are you so mad at him?" He said, "I cannot stand his constant recital. Even though he only comes in about once a month, it is exactly the same. If only he would tell me that he is feeling better! The best I ever get from him is a grudging acknowledgment that it is not as bad as it was." Such examples make up a very large part of the internist's medical practice; 40 percent of his patients, I would guess, are like this, and they occupy 60 percent of his time. But it is clear that his real exasperation centered on the fact that the patient would never give the doctor what the doctor wanted to hear: evidence of his therapeutic success.

For most physicians, the desire to succeed, to cure, to see patients improve is the real payoff. Doctors don't like to be losers, and as a result we tend to have a bad track record with the aged, with the alcoholic, with the drug users. These people are not, for many of us, very attractive because they do not fit our own personal rescue fantasies, our own great need to be successful and make people happier. For many years it has been my custom to teach medical students, internists, nurses, social workers one truism about gerontology: that you have to be satisfied with very small successes, with very small increments of improvement. If you are the kind of person who needs to see dramatic improvement, who needs to see development and recovery and great enhancement of function, then the field of aging and chronic illness is likely to be frustrating to you. The consequences of this overdeveloped therapeutic ambition, this need for the payoff, of the patient's saying "I am better," is reminiscent of a familiar phenomenon in many outpatient departments in general hospitals. The older patients with chronic illnesses are inclined to be referred back to the clinic at a time when somebody else will have to see them, not the original physician. Hence, there comes a self-fulfilling cycle: we don't want to see them, then they don't get better, and then because they don't get better we say, "you see you can't work with old people."

Seeing the Patient in the Broad Context

A last category of problems encountered with the aging might be described as those that arise from a failure to identify properly the patient or the problem in its entirety. More precisely, it is a kind of problem that arises from a failure to recognize that old age and the aging process are of such a nature that they must be seen in a broad context of family structure or even of community structure. This is an axiom of which social scientists and psychiatrists are only too cognizant; but the physician, accustomed to his familiar patient-doctor relationship, is likely to be somewhat oblivious to the axiom, unless he is truly alert to the implications of what being a family doctor really means.

Another illustration: the patient was a woman who had been under the care of her physician for a number of years, beginning in her middle sixties, and was treated for a number of gastrointestinal disturbances, largely functional in nature. She was responsive to the attentive care of the physician and particularly to the devotion and constant affection of her husband. They were a childless couple in retirement, living a life of what I would call faded gentility. He was studiously concerned about her welfare and equally concerned over maintaining the quality of life in which she manifested a certain gentle elegance and refinement, and which so characterized their life together. He was never complaining, not hysterically solicitous, but always appropriate in his feelings for his wife. Over the years, she became progressively demented, and as the first signs of her organic changes became evident, he was quick to make explanations for them to fill in the gaps of her own function, usually with very little in the way of complaint. He was always eager for reassurance that she would be all right. He seemed to take great comfort from the doctor's readiness to respond to her needs. Matters grew worse; she became quite confused, quite disoriented, could no longer be left by herself, and he was always by her side. Eventually, the situation declined to the point where she was putting the laundry in the oven, and in her confusion and deterioration became somewhat of a hazard. By this time they were into their seventies, their economic resources were largely depleted, and they had very little in the way of family that could be responsive. It was largely the husband who carried the burden of caring for her. Only through an event that clearly demonstrated the need for some intervention was it possible for the doctor to prevail upon him to consider placement in a home for the aged. He followed this recommendation, if not dutifully, at least with acceptance, cooperating with the staff of the facility which she entered.

Within days after she entered the facility, he appeared in the office of the social worker in charge of her admission and stated that he was going to kill himself as there was nothing to live for anymore. It was an extreme emergency and the authenticity of his statements and of his behavior required immediate response; accordingly, I arranged for him to be admitted to a psychiatric hospital. The course in the hospital was unbelievable. This man who had for many years functioned in a remarkably adaptive way, sustaining the burden of his wife's long period of illness and decline, broke down and deteriorated himself. He lapsed into a constant type of hypochondriasis, developed physical disabilities of an extremely regressive nature, was totally unable to care for himself, and required urgent admission to the very same facility to which his wife had been admitted.

This is by no means, of course, an unfamiliar story. What strikes me about it is that the physician who had looked after his wife for many years had continued to count on the husband to sustain the separation and loss of his wife as he had sustained other losses in the past. In retrospect, I could say that during the last year or two of the wife's decline, the real patient was the husband, not the wife. What could be done for her was clearly evident long before; what was necessary for him was somehow overlooked largely because he didn't speak of his own needs until the very end, when he spoke of them so graphically. I do not consider this an example of neglect or really of failure on the part of the doctor. I think the omission arose from the physician's traditional posture of dealing with the patient in the classical model and not seeing the problems of aging in their broadest social or familial context. Something similar often occurs within a larger community when situations involving the aged who have deteriorated and declined to the point where they become subjects for intervention by the public health authorities are allowed to go on because everyone sees the problem but no one feels empowered to intervene.

Physician Failure at Protective Intervention

I do not at this time wish to enter into a full discussion of the problems of protective intervention in the aged nor into a discussion of problems of self-determinism in work with the aged. I would only say in no other field is the physician called upon to intervene in this way, a role for which he or she is not equipped, is ill-educated, and is reluctant to assume. The frequency with which illness, decline, and deterioration in a parent will set off a chain reaction of breakdown in a child or a spouse is all too evident. It is equally apparent to physicians, but they are loath to take the aggressive intervention posture that is frequently called for. Particularly this is true when the situation demands intervention such as protective placement and where the physician is inclined to throw it back into the hands of the family. Physicians, it is true, are very ready to tell the family that it is necessary to seek placement, but they are not ready to make the further effort to support the family in seeking information about placement or see them through the ordeal of making arrangements.

It is always striking to me to be called by distinguished and knowledgeable physicians who will simply ask me what nursing home I recommend. I am always impressed by their own failure to find out for themselves. These are devoted, dedicated physicians, yet they keep themselves in ignorance of the wide spectrum of social service agencies, information agencies, and other facilities designed to help them with precisely this problem. I think this phenomenon is only one more version of the failure of the medical profession to enter into the serious exploration of the entire gerontological science, as can best be attested to by the long delays in generating teaching and service programs within university and medical school curricula. That such developments are now blossoming all around us is of course highly commendable. Although universities today are embracing the field, the embrace seems to me to be often still tentative and hesitant in nature. This is progress. Twenty years ago aging usually evoked bland indifference. How to overcome that indifference is the topic of this book.

PART IV
PHYSICIAN
CHARACTERISTICS

The second source of difficulty in establishing a successful doctor-elderly patient relationship has been identified as relating to physician characteristics, the subject of this section. The risk of "blaming the doctor," like the risk of "blaming the patient," is avoided by the gerontologist and the psychiatrist who contribute here. Physician features, although the main topic, are considered in the context of patient characteristics as well. As in the prior section, the interplay is highlighted.

Dr. Marshall selects for elaboration three aspects of relations between practitioners and patients: authority relations, affective relations, and issues of therapeutic activism. Physician characteristics have differential impacts in each of these areas: physicians' religious beliefs and lower-social-class origin, for example, are two characteristics related to therapeutic activism. Older general practitioners, despite their longer experience, tend to be least knowledgeable about aging and disease. They may also be less familiar with high technology medicine, which in turn relates to area of specialization. Specialist adherents of the most modern technological advances often favor active therapeutic intervention with dramatic results, and are less interested in the chronically ill and elderly. Thus, elderly physicians may be the ones left to treat the aged, although they are not necessarily the best equipped to do so.

Marshall develops the reciprocal effects of authority and affectivity in an innovative way. He notes that patients seek respect. It is not necessary for a physician to like his or her patients, but the patients must feel they are respected. Indeed, practitioners' authority in the biomedical sphere of patient care depends at least in part on respect in the social sphere. However, this gerontologist warns against identifying the psychosocial concerns of the patient as falling within the physician's mandate and responsibility. Such attempts at medicalization of areas in which most practitioners' expertise is uncertain can be considered invasive by patients. Authority relations are essentially power relations, Marshall explains, which is one clue to the problem of noncompliance. In the strain for control of the situation in dealing with an illness, patients can retain power over their lives by failing to comply with physician regimen. Such an act of "medical sabotage" may even be a source of patient self-respect.

Noting the brevity of most interaction between physicians and patients, a few hours a year, Marshall suggests that the setting for the interaction may be more important than physician characteristics in influencing the effectiveness of elderly patients' care. However, he urges that one often-neglected characteristic be considered, and that is the sociohistorical period experienced by the health provider. The cohort effect, related as it is to age, can be one element in the phenomenon of "burn out."

Dr. Breslau's chapter addresses burn out, a sense of weariness and inadequacy in dealing with the elderly, in illuminating detail. The loss of a therapeutic viewpoint is due to the health care team's taking on the patient's sense of hopelessness and discouragement when faced with catastrophic illness in the elderly. Physicians then tend to fall back on four fallacies, or rationalizations for their inactivity or desire to rid themselves of the patient. The custodial fallacy involves inappropriate recommendation of institutionalization; the specialist fallacy permits deflecting the patient's care through referral. The uncooperative patient fallacy is based on the belief that physicians should control the relationship. Like Marshall, Breslau sees noncompliance as a way for patients to restore their own control. Finally, the family responsibility fallacy relates to attempts to place the burden of care on the family, on the grounds that the patient is beyond medical help, when in fact the physician, distressed by the situation, has lost a treatment perspective.

Two revealing clinical histories are presented, illustrating the process by which an impasse occurs, when a patient's attitude of helplessness and sense of loss is transmitted to the physician, who, in an attempt to relieve his feelings, loses the therapeutic viewpoint.

The need for physicians to understand the psychological mechanisms at work in order to deal with them is stressed in the chapter. Breslau argues that caregivers must learn to consider their own reactions as an integal part of the patient's illness. He shows how this approach was successful in dealing with a particularly difficult case of an aged diabetic woman. Not all elderly present these types of problems, although those who do may take up a disproportionafe amount of a physician's time. Consequently, Breslau considers it essential that a systematic approach to dealing with negative therapeutic relationships in geriatric care be developed and that this must involve training primary care doctors to think in psychological terms.

Although the aging of the physician is discussed, neither chapter alludes to the situation where the patient outlives the physician he or she may have been using for several years or where the patient relocates and must find a new source of care. The resulting discontinuity and likely difficulty in establishing a new relationship could have negative effects for the health of the elderly individual, and may not necessarily be a rare occurrence. Relocation to a new community or better climate, as a voluntary act, will involve prior recognition that a new relationship needs to be established and will be less distressing than the death of one's "regular doctor." This is an event that the old-old, the increasing numbers in their eighties and nineties, will almost certainly have to face. Dealing with interrupted doctor-patient relationships as a result of practitioner mortality is a problem, perhaps not unique but certainly not uncommon, for the elderly. It is probable that a technology for helping the older person cope with the loss of a physician and deal with finding a new one may be developed, once the existence of this problem area is recognized.

9
Physician Characteristics and Relationships with Older Patients*

VICTOR W. MARSHALL, Ph.D.

Innumerable aspects of the relationship between patients and doctors are of potential practical and theoretical interest. In this chapter I circumscribe this vast topic by focusing on three aspects of the doctor-patient relationship that are of central importance for older people, largely ignoring a host of factors that condition or qualify these aspects. Further, by paying special attention to physician characteristics that affect the doctor-patient relationship, patient and setting characteristics and the interaction process between patient and physician receive less attention than they might.[1]

The three aspects of the doctor-patient relationship I have selected are:

1. the authority relationship,
2. the affective relationship, and
3. the issue of therapeutic activism, or the extent to which the physician aggressively seeks cure.

This review is, therefore, highly selective, and may be thought of as an essay highly critical of predominant conceptualizations of the relationship be-

*Because this is a recent area of interest for me, I have drawn heavily on colleagues for advice and criticism. In addition to other contributors to this volume, I would like especially to thank Susan French, Joanne Gard Marshall, Carolyn Rosenthal, and David Sackett of McMaster University; Merrijoy Kelner and Oswald Hall of the University of Toronto; Linda Breytspraak of the University of Missouri-Kansas City; Rodney Coe of St. Louis University; Neena Chappell of the University of Manitoba; Ingrid Connidis of the University of Western Ontario; A. S. Macpherson of McGill University; and Joseph Tindale of York University. This essay draws theoretically on collaborative work with Rosenthal, Macpherson, and French on the nurse-patient-family relationship. My work has been enabled by research support as a National Health Scientist under grant 6606–1568–48 from Health and Welfare Canada.

tween physicians and patients and an attempt to point to promising areas for future research.

Discussing the authority relationship allows some critical thinking about models of the doctor-patient relationship, including models of the sick role, in terms of their applicability to older patients. In my view, the most important single aspect of the doctor-patient relationship is the vast authority differential between the patient and the doctor, yet conceptualizations of this differential have on the whole failed to treat authority as a social process.

In the section on the affective relationship, I argue that although on the whole, doctors do not like older patients, this probably does not matter a great deal. Physician attitudes vary greatly contemporaneously and over historical periods, and the relationship between attitudes and actions is not necessarily strong in any abstract sense.

If there is an aspect of the doctor-patient relationship wherein attitudes are significant in their effects, it is probably in the conceptions held by doctors of the relationship between aging and disease and of the value of actively attempting to make older patients well. This is discussed in the section on therapeutic activism.

Before turning to the three aspects of the doctor-patient relationship, I discuss some general features of that relationship and some problems in trying to understand it.

What Doctor-Patient Relationship?

For all the concern about the doctor-patient relationship, we must bear in mind that this relationship is usually tenuous. If measured by frequency of interaction, the relationship is not strong, even for older people, who see physicians much more often than do younger people. If measured by duration of each interactional episode, the data on average length of a physician visit (reported elsewhere in this book) suggest that even for older patients, whose visits are of longer duration, there is little time for a strong bond to develop between patient and doctor. Even 8–10 visits per year to a general practitioner or family physician, with an average of about 15 minutes per visit, implies that the relationship has perhaps 2 hours per year in which to flourish. In the primary care situation, patients and their doctors may grow old together, and over the years they might have spent as much as a few days together at most. The hospitalized patient spends very little time copresent with a doctor, the bulk of hospital care being given not by doctors but by nurses.

Although I will not abandon the term relationship to describe something linking a patient and a doctor, serious consideration should be given to directing research toward analysis of doctor-patient encounters or interactional episodes that may or may not lead to relationships of any duration or strength.[2] When there does exist a relationship between the doctor and the patient, analysis is complicated by virtue of the fact that relationships are not static. The many properties that characterize such relationships change over time (Bloor & Horobin, 1975:280). The relationship is, therefore, ideally described as a process rather than as a state.

This process is shaped in some measure by the course of the disease or physiological state of the patient (a biological factor) and by the course of the illness (the definition given by the patient to the disease). It is also shaped by the application of medical technology and other behavioral initiatives by the physician. I argue that emphasis should be given in future research to the interactional strategies employed by patients and their doctors as they negotiate the many properties of their relationship and that the relationship be conceptualized as a career in the general sociological sense of that term (Becker & Strauss, 1956; Hughes, 1971; Marshall, 1978-79).

Viewing the doctor-patient relationship as a career considers it as a complex interactive process that unfolds in a situation with at least the potential for negotiation or bargaining between the two key parties and other secondary parties affiliated to them (nurses, families, hospital administrators, etc.). Doctor-patient interaction is not a two-person drama. The interaction between doctor and patient is not usually simply diadic. Health professionals, administrators, insurance companies, family, and friends often get into the act both as contingent players and as intermediaries in the dramas that unfold.

Since Henderson described physician-patient relationships as a social system (1935), a variety of models has been formulated to describe the complex of relations between doctors and patients. Some of the better-known models have been formulated, recast, or criticized by contributors to this book (Bloom, 1965; Bloom & Summey, 1978; Wilson & Bloom, 1972; Engel, 1977b).

Coe (1970:103) has suggested the inappropriateness of assuming a great sharing of expectations between physician and patient, especially in the case of chronic illness, and he questions the assumption, made in the Parsonian model, for example, of a strain toward equilibrium in the doctor-patient relationship. Coe notes the importance of communication and the authority imbalance between doctor and patient (1970:97-8, 104). These suggest a much more dynamic relational process through which doctor and patient negotiate the course of their relationship over time. However, most studies of the doctor-patient relationship focus not on process but on attributes of either doctor or patient that affect their relationship. A prime example is research on compliance with medical regimens, which tends to focus unduly on patient characteristics affecting compliance; a good example is "blaming the victim" (Ryan, 1971). On the other hand, quality-of-care research tends to ignore the patient and focus on properties of the physician and the practice setting. Both approaches convey an image of greater stability than is warranted.

The general literature on these matters is voluminous, but empirical or even theoretical treatment of aged patients or of age variability in patients is almost entirely absent. Patterns must be induced from many studies that do not stand too solidly on their own, often with a commonsensical extension to find relevance for the aged patient. Aged patients are not a species set apart from humanity, however, and my approach has been to focus on issues that are important for patients of all ages but perhaps accentuated in importance in the later years.

As I critically review the three analytical dimensions of the doctor-patient relationship, I attempt to assess the importance of physician characteristics, to identify ambiguities and gaps in our knowledge, and to recommend research priorities.

The Negotiation of Authority and Deference

Authority is a social relationship (rather than an attribute), in which one party gives legitimacy to another in matters of mutual concern. If one party acts in a way that has consequences for another without the assent of the other, this is brute power. Authority is legitimate power. Legitimacy, in turn, may be conferred on the basis of a number of criteria (Haug, 1978). Most models of the doctor-patient relationship (Engel, 1977b; Friedson, 1970b, 1970c; Parsons, 1951; Szasz & Hollender, 1956) focus on the authority of expertise based on the physician's exclusive monopoly of knowledge, but there are other bases upon which patients give authority to doctors. Deference given to doctors may have a basis in traditional authority relationships between social classes (Haug, 1978). Doctors have rational-legal authority, or the authority of bureaucratic office, in being legally mandated to act in certain ways toward patients (French & Raven, 1959; Haug, 1978). If a doctor's authority is challenged, a reply might be made on the basis of expertise, on the basis of "this is the way it is and always has been," or on the basis of "the rules."

Doctors are usually presumed to have authority over patients, but authority can also be given to the patient by the doctor. Thus, in one model of mutual participation described by Szasz and Hollender (1956), ". . . the greater the intellectual, educational, and general experiential similarity between physician and patient, the more appropriate and necessary this model of therapy becomes." This formulation seems patronizingly to argue that if the patients can only be a lot like doctors, they should be given the right to run their own affairs. But it has also been argued that greater mutual participation, or a yielding of authority by the physician to the patient, is called for in the case of chronic illness, where the patient ideally becomes highly active in his or her own care.

Authority is given by one party to another in a relationship. However, it is not *a* given, but rather the focus of negotiation between patient and doctor. Roth (1972) provides a framework for viewing the negotiation of authority through his concept of control actions:

> Control actions are not carefully thought out and preplanned. . . . Rather, the contol actions typically arise in situational negotiations. Each party to the negotiation reacts to the behavior of the other in a way that he believes will tend to keep the choice or initiative in his hands. . . .

From this perspective, authority is a negotiated seizing and yielding of control over the course of treatment and over other aspects of the relationship between physician and patient.

Authority in the Biomedical and Psychosocial Spheres

A host of studies have shown that patients want two things from their doctors: they want technical competence in treatment, and they want respect and treatment as people. The latter is often found to be listed as of greater importance than technical competency (Cartwright, 1967:21; Ben-Sira, 1976; Congalton, 1969; Reader, Pratt, & Mudd, 1957). This may be because technical competency is taken for granted by patients. When patients want technical competency, they are asking the doctor to operate within a traditional biomedical model. In this model, the doctor brings medical knowledge and technology to bear in treating, not a patient, but a disease. The patient is passive, and complies with regimens of treatment administered and prescribed by the doctor (Wilson & Bloom, 1972; Szasz & Hollender, 1956).

Most patients are willing to give the physician authority in traditional aspects of the doctor-patient relationship when activities are focused in the biomedical sphere. However, life is not so simple, and most patients expect more than biomedical intervention in their disease.[3] Older patients, especially, want a delimited but qualitatively different intervention at the psychosocial level (Cartwright, 1967:21–24). I stress delimited, because the evidence, sparse though it is, does not suggest that the patient is anxious to surrender personhood to the care of a physician.

In the application of biomedical technology to a disease of the body, the control initiatives of the patient are severely constrained by the patient's lack of expert knowledge. Here we have the ascendancy of expert authority.[4] However, in the other highly valued aspects of the doctor-patient relationship, the knowledge disparity is not so great as when considering biomedical aspects of the disease. Sorenson (1974) has argued:

> . . . we should not expect the varieties of doctor-patient interactions that occur in modern medicine to be described by a single power-dependency arrangement. Medicine as a field of applied knowledge varies significantly from one health issue to another; there is more or less certainty about various health matters, and we should expect to find corresponding shifts in the types of doctor-patient encounters as health issues change. [Sorenson, 1974:366]

Sorenson (1974) posits that the patient is more likely to be involved in clinical decision making in areas of uncertainty such as when new technological developments are introduced in medicine or when previously nonmedical areas (e.g., genetic counseling) are brought under medical domination. Similarly, Fox (1959) reports a highly collegial relationship between doctors and patients on the experimental ward she studied (discussed in Sorenson, 1974, and Eisenberg, 1979). Attention to the psychological and social aspects of the patient is precisely such an uncertainty area. The technology of psychosocial care is new—to the doctor in any case —and its application is an expansion of the role of the doctor—a medicalization of nonmedical aspects of social life. As such, the situation of psychosocial care requires greater patient collaboration and also a lessening of hierarchical boundaries between physician and patient.

Psychosocial care is coming into its own as a generally applauded approach to the care of patients at all ages. It may be of even greater importance in the care of the aged because of the presence of multiple diseases, the overlay of acute or chronic conditions, the lack of alternatives to professionally delivered social support caused by the social isolation of many older patients, and the increased importance of caring rather than curing in older patients for whom, often, nothing can be done except to give care.

Enlightened clinicians, medical sociologists, and health scientists may be inclined to abandon a traditional biomedical model for a new, psychosocially oriented model, but patients have not been so inclined. Rather, they seem to suspect that psychosocial care (this is not a language patients use) is secondary when it comes to the crunch. When they are ill, they want to be made well (or, if not that, they want to be made comfortable), and it is in medical technology and not psychosocial care that they put their faith.

Within this order of priorities, however, patients—and, seemingly, older patients especially—want to be treated with respect. Respect is a term relevant in a vastly different model of the doctor-patient relationship, a model in which both doctor and patient are viewed as persons, and in which what goes on between them is viewed as interaction instead of the action of the one on something the other has. Psychosocial care can be carried to the point where it is invasive of the territorial self of the patient.

Haug and Sussman (1969), discussing the "revolt of the client" against professional authority, state these concerns as follows:

> The slogan for all groups is, "don't call me, I'll call you." The client seems to be rejecting what he considers meddling under the cover of professional concern. Outreach programs from the client perspective have become "out-grab." . . . The "whole man" approach in medicine infringes on areas of social relations where clients consider themselves competent; patients want to turn to the doctor when in trouble, but not to be bothered otherwise. This suggests that the client is demanding the right to define the problem and then call upon the professional only as a specialist in a narrow domain. [Haug & Sussman, 1969:157–158]

In summary, the kind of authority that the patient will give to the physician differs according to the biomedical or psychosocial nature of the problem. Expert authority is quite freely given because of the knowledge or competence gap between physician and patient. This is a gap that is even wider for older patients than younger ones—a point on which I will expand below. Patients want more than technically good care, however. They want considerate treatment as human beings. Psychosocial care as a newly emerging health technology does not provide such consideration in any automatic way, because patients may fear that the clinician is moving too broadly into areas considered to be private or none of the physician's business.

Compliance

I now want to argue that the expert authority assigned to the physician is itself precarious and contingent in some measure on patients being satisfied that the physician is treating them with respect.

One indicator of the willingness of patients to accept the authority of doctors, in the traditional biomedical model of the doctor-patient relationship, is compliance with prescribed therapeutic regimens (Haug & Lavin,

1978). This is not, however, a terribly strong indicator because compliance is affected by so many factors other than authority attributed to the physician (this literature is assessed in Haynes, Sackett, & Taylor, 1979).

The rationality of compliance is a direct function of the soundness of medical advice. Physicians vary in their treatments and their advice. Their treatments sometimes cause or risk causing iatrogenic illness, and their advice is at times bad. An obvious example is the tendency of some physicians to prescribe antidepressants too readily to women and to the elderly (most of whom also happen to be women). Variability on this dimension intersects with therapeutic activism, but is in some degree independent of it.

What physician characteristics are associated with variability in drug prescription? There is some evidence that doctors who are subject to peer review may be more cautious in their prescribing habits (Wolfe, 1974:57; Wolfe & Badgley, 1973:60–67). On the whole, these tend to be younger doctors. British data show that older doctors are more likely to rely on drug company representatives and mailings for information about their drugs (Wilson et al., 1964, cited in Wolfe & Badgley, 1973:62). A Swedish study (Lilja, 1976) found that younger doctors gave more weight to cost and to side effects of drugs in making a selection than did older doctors, who focused more on the curing effect of the drug. In one of two hypothetical cases, older doctors differed more than younger ones from the judgments of an expert panel in their selection of a drug. These differences were not, however, great. Dunnell and A. Cartwright (1972; A. Cartwright, 1974) found that doctors thought they would prescribe less if they had to spend longer in their consultations with patients; however, they also found higher prescription assignment on the part of physicians with relatively few patients. It is possible that more conditions are discovered in the longer time period, leading to elevated prescription rates.

Patients may feel satisfied when they receive a prescription from the doctor, believing that something concrete is being done; however, physicians are more satisfied with consultations the fewer prescriptions they give (Balint, 1972:107–108; A. Cartwright, 1974). If patients come to the doctor in effect asking for a drug, then whether or not they get one might reflect their ability to negotiate. Dunnell and A. Cartwright (1972) found that, when controlling for symptomatology, middle-class patients were assigned more prescriptions than lower-class patients, possibly reflecting their differential negotiating ability (A. Cartwright, 1974).

Stimson (1978) has shown how the physician may give in to patient requests for drugs as a device to manipulate other aspects of the relationship. A two-week prescription for a drug known by the doctor to be inefficacious may secure a return visit to obtain a renewal of the prescription. Giving in to the patient regarding the drug is, thus, a kind of currency exchanged for other valued behavior such as continuity of care. Beyond this, however, Davis (1971) reports that good compliance is associated with the doctor's offering considerable explanation in a situation of positive affect in the clinical encounter. Compliance was found to be low when the doctor asked for information without giving feedback.

What other physician characteristics are associated with compliance? In research by the Kaiser-Permanente group (Hurtado, Greenlick, & Colombo, 1973), it was found that the appointment failure rate was slightly lower in the case of older physicians. This finding, the authors assert, "probably resulted because older physicians tend to have a long-standing caseload fostering a close physician-patient relationship." This explanation is more plausible in the light of lower failure rates with increasing tenure of physician appointment. Both factors may, however, involve physicians dropping patients from their practice who do not keep appointments. In that study, which of course refers to only a limited aspect of compliance, compliance was unaffected by other physician variables such as country of training, whether or not the physician had administrative responsibility, and how many patients were carried by the physician.

In her British study, A. Cartwright (1967:112) concludes that both patients and doctors prefer to have a relationship that is closer and warmer than the "affectively neutral" relationship described by Parsons (1951:434). The general pattern is that compliance is enhanced by departure from a purely technical relationship. Thus, for example, Geertsen, Gray, and Ward (1973) found 61 percent full compliers among arthritic patients in their sample who perceived the doctor to be "personal," compared to only 35 percent full compliance in those who characterized the relationship as more "businesslike." Full compliance was clinic attendance and fulfilling medication instructions as rated by doctors, in this study.[5]

Hoenig and Ragg (1966) found that appointments made with a specific clinician rather than with a clinic enhanced rates of compliance or adherence in the case of psychiatric outpatients. Whether this applies with equal force to other patients who might not value a personalized or comprehensive relationship so much is unclear.

The list of factors enhancing adherence to medical regimens turns out to be a breakdown of factors that individualize and personalize the doctor-patient relationship: having a personal appointment, having known the doctor for a longer period of time, perceiving the doctor as personal and interested rather than as businesslike, having a doctor who explains the illness and treatment regimen in some detail.

What do you do if you are not terribly sure you are being given the best advice or treatment by your physician? You may look for another physician or fail to come back for the next appointment, or partially or totally ignore his or her instructions. It is, in fact, not terribly easy to switch doctors (Haug, 1978; A. Cartwright, 1967:18–20; Gill, 1978). Motivation and trust are important factors in compliance, and they seem to be based largely on satisfaction with the interpersonal or psychosocial aspects of the encounter.

This reading of the data is heavily influenced by British studies, where the delivery system is quite different and where social class differences between patients and physicians are perhaps greater than in the United States and some other countries (Haug, 1976; Mechanic, 1972). Nonetheless, with older patients we are in general dealing with a social relationship between a high-status, well-educated doctor and a lower-status, economically insecure, and ill-educated patient. Often, the authority contrast is heightened because most doctors are male and most older patients are female.

Many patient, physician, and organizational features affect compliance. One additional major reason for noncompliance may be the patient's attempt to protect a little integrity in a kind of class conflict with the physician. Noncompliance is perhaps in some respects akin to industrial sabotage or work to rule. The employee knows he or she needs the job, but stopping the line for a while might be needed, too, as a relief from machine-paced work. Working to rule is a kind of holding back of one's entire personhood from the role of worker. Noncompliance, or failure to fully adhere to clinical regimens, might be considered as analogous: a kind of role-distancing behavior in which the patient asserts individuality and gives at least partial resistance to the constraints of the patient role, while at the same time in effect making a claim to some personal control over aspects of the doctor-patient relationship.

Conflict and Negotiation

The authority relationship between patients and doctors is realized through their consultations. Any analysis of authority in the doctor-patient relationship should take cognizance of Stimson's advice (1978:77) that "it is useful to view the outcome of the consultation as a result of negotiation or bargaining between patient and doctor, rather than as a simple product of the application of the doctor's knowledge and skills to the patient's problems."

In such bargaining, the patient is at a distinct disadvantage compared to the doctor because of a lack of expert knowledge and because of traditional deference patterns between the social classes. With older patients, these differences are only exacerbated because of the lower educational

levels of most old people, because of their generally lower-social-class origins, and because of the fact that a very large proportion of them have been
downwardly mobile if measured by level of income. In short, if life-long
characteristics set the patient apart from the doctor, aging only increases
such differences. The older patient has, therefore, little hope of great success in negotiation attempts with doctors.

Haug's (1979) findings support this view. In her survey of attitudes toward physician authority in a Midwestern state, she found a general reluctance to challenge physician authority, but persons under the age of 60
were three times as likely as persons over age 60 to attain highest scores
on willingness to challenge physician authority.[6] Older persons were also, despite a longer history of health care, somewhat less likely to report having behaved in a challenging way, such as by secretly obtaining a second opinion, changing doctors, or telling them their advice
was not satisfactory.

Stimson has argued that within the doctor-patient encounter conflict is down-played:

> The relative position of patient and doctor can be summed up as the
> *idealization of ignorance*. While the patient may not necesarily feel ignorant
> (or even perceive the doctor to be omniscient) and the doctor may be aware
> that his knowledge is limited, ignorance and knowledge are idealized. . . .
> Doctors and patients act towards each other as though they personified these
> opposite attributes. . . . both patient and doctor collude in setting a scene in
> which the doctor can 'act like a doctor' and the patient 'act like a patient.'
> [Stimson, 1978:79; see also Danziger, 1978]

Stimson says that the patient uses only "devious strategies" to try to
influence the doctor, and argues that the patient's presentation of him- or
herself as ignorant only serves to reinforce the doctor's ideological stance
that, indeed, the profession has a monopoly on medical knowledge. Older
patients, thus, seem more ready than younger patients to grant this monopoly.

The interpretation I have been developing focuses on the interaction
in the doctor-patient relationship, as each party seeks to negotiate and
bargain in his or her own interests. This approach draws on conflict theory
and the negotiated order approach in sociology.[7] From this perspective,
the question of authority in the doctor-patient relationship becomes recast into the questions: what factors variably affect the bargaining
strength of each party, and how do these parties bargain with one another over time?

Recall that in the Kaiser-Permanente study (Hurtado, Greenlick, &
Colombo, 1973), compliance was unaffected by country of training and

whether or not the physician had administrative responsibility. These factors can be viewed as variables affecting the authority of expertise and of office. Here, and in other studies, such authority seems less important than that which comes from the development of a personal relationship in securing compliance. The authority of the physician within the biomedical sphere is contingent on the lessening of authority differences in the psychosocial sphere.

In her British interviews with doctors and other officials in the health service, Haug found a persistence of charismatic authority, but this appeared to be decreasing with successive cohorts of physicians. As she says, "Notably, it was the younger doctors and medical student interviewees who most expressed the desire to rid themselves of any charismatic aura, who seemed to feel strongly that their role should be demystified" (Haug, 1978:247).

Beyond a willingness to share power with the patient and to form a doctor-patient relationship that encompasses more than purely technical biomedical aspects, other factors may enter as resources available to the doctor in negotiating the shape of the doctor-patient relationship with the older patient. These include the doctor's knowledge, beliefs, and attitudes toward older patients and older people in general; the ability of the doctor to cope with stresses likely to be encountered in such care; and the values placed on and received from giving chronic and acute care to older patients.

The Affective Relationship between Patient and Physician

It is unfortunately true that many doctors do not like to care for older patients. I believe that this is not something peculiar to physicians and that it is not something that can be greatly changed. Rather, the delivery of health care ought to be organized so that this unfortunate fact has few consequences.

In a British study reported as long ago as 1967, A. Cartwright found that only 4 percent of general practitioners listed geriatrics as a special interest. Geriatrics has developed greatly since that time in Great Britain, but it is just beginning to gain in importance in North America. Why should interest in caring for the older patient be so low?

In a classic article, Kastenbaum (1964) reviewed four reasons why psychotherapists might be reluctant to deal with older patients. These reasons are probably generalizable to other kinds of doctor-patient encounter. He argues (1964:140): " . . . it would seem that the conscientious psychotherapist might reasonably be expected to hesitate a moment before offering his services to an aged person. He feels a realistic need for more experience and systematic knowledge." Additional reasons are the possible status-contamination of caring for clientele who are largely lower-class; the fact that the pain, deterioration, and proximity to death of the aged might be taken as foreshadowing the fate of the therapist; and a cost-benefits argument that work with the young yields greater dividends in years of healthy life than does care of the old" (see also Karasu, Stein, & Charles, 1979).

Lasagna (1969:62) remarks that physicians find little pleasure in chronic care, and there is evidence for this in the use of the terms "crock," "turkey," and "gomer" to designate chronic patients and those whose care has high psychosocial and low physical components (Mumford, 1970:208; Reynolds & Bice, 1971). Mumford (1970:208) found 70 percent of house staff in large medical-school-affiliated hospitals, but only a little over 50 percent of those in smaller community hospitals, preferring a patient whose illness is entirely physical. Since chronic care has large non-physical components, and since it is increasingly evident in older patients, this suggests an incompatability between physicians who practice high-technology medicine and the care of older chronic patients. This was rather dramatically illustrated in Mumford's intensive study of a community and a university hospital. She found that three-fourths of the physician repondents in the former hospital but none of those in the latter hospital said they attached "great importance" to ability to establish rapport with patients (Mumford, 1970:187).

Attitudes toward older patients are, therefore, related to styles of practice and the therapeutic orientation of the physician. As Eisdorfer (1973) remarks, " . . . the aged patient's use of the physician as a confidant often runs counter to the expectations of today's practitioner, who sees himself primarily as a specialist in the practice of scientific medicine." Such doctors are likely to attribute triviality to a high proportion of the presenting complaints brought to them, and are not likely to take seriously the patient's bargaining attempts in their encounter (Gough, 1977).

Hornung and Massagli (1979) point out that although patients are better able to judge their doctors on affective qualities than on technical competence, doctors are socialized to emphasize the latter. In a study of physicians in Maryland, they found a strong correlation between a doctor's tendency to define a patient's symptoms as "hypochondriacal" and as a "challenge to clinical competence and professional integrity." One causal chain is highly relevant in the case of older patients, who prefer to spend more time with the physician than the physician frequently wishes to give. They argue that " . . . patients who disrupt the physician's schedule by using more time than the physician had planned to spend diagnosing and treating them are most likely to elicit a definition of hypochondriasis and subsequently a definition of their behavior as representing a challenge to the physician's integrity and judgment." To the extent that this is true, it might account in great measure for the physician tendency to dislike older patients.

Physicians in this study did vary in their tendency to make such characterizations, but the physician characteristics studied (e.g., board certification, country of medical education) were correlated with setting characteristics such as solo versus group practice, to which the authors assign greater importance.

Within one type of practice setting, the outpatient clinic, Sussman and associates (1967) distinguished between physicians who are patient-care oriented and those who are profession oriented. To the profession-oriented doctors, it made little difference in their work satisfaction whether they worked with chronic or acute patients; however, patient-care-oriented doctors were more satisfied to work with acute patients, because they valued attaining a positive outcome (Sussman et al., 1967:134). These authors conclude that:

> . . . staff members who enjoy a challenge and like to interact with a patient who is well informed about his illness will usually prefer to treat the chronically ill, who are believed to have these characteristics. But those who are gratified by an independent patient who helps himself to recover, manages better for himself while cooperating with treatment, and who provides the satisfaction of showing improvement, will usually prefer to treat the acutely ill. [Sussman et. al., 1967:136]

Some variability in this range of attitudes has been found by age. Ford and associates (1967:138) found middle-aged and older doctors in Cleveland more favorable to older patients than younger doctors; Davis (1968) found that junior doctors (interns) expressed more concern over interpersonal relations with their patients and that senior doctors professed more sympathy for them.

Overall, however, the relationship between demographic characteristics and attitudes toward the aged, toward chronic care, or toward psychosocial care is likely quite unimportant in relation to the behavioral aspects of such care, which are more conditioned by work experience and the practice setting. Thus, psychiatrists with extensive work experience with the aged have been found to have more positive feelings toward older patients than psychiatrists with little such experience (Cyrus-Lutz & Gaitz, 1972). Older psychiatrists were more likely to stress the intelligence and wisdom of old people, while younger psychiatrists stressed their appreciativeness.

Although there is undoubtedly some selection by physicians to practice in settings in keeping with their own stance toward older patients, chronic care, and psychosocial care, the setting itself appears to have a major impact on the relationship that can develop between older patient and physician. Relevant setting characteristics in hospital, clinic, or primary care are the degree of emphasis on high-technology medicine; appointment arrangements; solo, group, or team practice arrangements; and billing by service unit or by time.

Given the pervasiveness of negative attitudes toward care of the elderly, it is important to consider the possibility that doctors can be either selected or socialized to want to give the kind of care we need for older people.

Attempts to develop attitudes in medical students that are favorable to caring for older patients have not been very successful. Spence and associates (1968) found no difference between first- and fourth-year medical students in strongly negative attitudes toward the elderly. A review of the literature on attempts to change attitudes in medical school found that attempts to reinforce humanistic and holistic attitudes among students have, at best, short-lived effects (Rezler, 1974; for one reported exception, see Poole & Sanson-Fisher, 1979).

Research on the attitudes and career choices of successive cohorts of Harvard medical students challenges the conventional wisdom that socialization makes a significant difference in attitudes and behavior (Funkenstein, 1978). Most of the variance in career choice and in preferred age of patients could best be explained by the general sociohistorical characteristics of the period through which the students had lived, rather than by either socialization or background (selection) variables. For example, during the 1940s and most of the 1950s, there was a great emphasis on specialization in medical care. "Positive attitudes were toward the young and those with clear-cut physical illnesses. Negative attitudes were toward the elderly and those with psychological symptoms" (Funkenstien, 1978:18). The following 10 years evidenced attention to scientific and academic medicine, with a majority of students still reacting negatively toward older patients. A brief era of student activism from 1969–1970 drew many applicants from the social sciences, and medical students became more concerned with issues of health care delivery. "This time, students reacted positively to the elderly and to those with psychological problems and negatively to the affluent" (Funkenstein, 1978:23). The period 1971–1974 was highly competitive because of the larger number of applicants produced by the baby boom cohort, and attitudes swung back toward favoring younger over older patients and clear-cut physical illnesses over psychological distress. However, as governmental programs led to increased career opportunities in primary care in the mid-1970s, attitudes toward the older patient improved again. By the late 1970s, 48 percent of these Harvard students expressed positive attitudes toward working with older patients; however, negative attitudes continued to be strong toward those with psychological problems (Funkenstein, 1978:33). Coe, Pepper, and Mattis (1977) report very similar results in a study of several cohorts of medical students at St. Louis University.

The morals of this story are: that attitudes toward the aged go up and down, but this reflects broader societal patterns and has little to do with the health care system per se or with medical education; and that behavior is affected by an opportunity structure more than by an attitudinal structure. If money is put into postdoctoral awards and clinical positions and programs for the elderly, people will be attracted to these positions if the job market is tight enough. We are likely to accomplish a great deal more for the elderly by mandating organizational structures and delivery systems that will serve them than by trying to shape attitudes. Therefore, in some senses, it is not useful to focus unduly on the negative attitudes toward the elderly that are held by many people in general in our society, including doctors.

There is also another moral, a methodological one. The various studies of attitudes toward the older patient that have been done over the years in the United States and other nations might, in fact, tell us little about the relationships between various physician characteristics in general and such attitudes in general. Instead, they may tell us only about the attitudes of that cohort in a particular historical era.[8] The methodological lesson for us in this has been made by C. Wright Mills: that we need to be concerned with the intersection of biography and history, of private troubles and public issues, and any explanation based solely on individual characteristics is bound to be distorting. This is not to deny the importance of attitudes entirely but only to urge caution in interpreting the relationship between attitudes and behavior. If an attitude defines a reward that will dispose an individual to behave in a given way, the existence of the reward is a function not of the individual but of the opportunity structure of the environment.[9]

Stress and Burnout in the Doctor

In recent years, increasing attention has been given to a different perspective on the affective relationship between doctors and patients, in focusing on the emotional consequences of giving such care for the clinician. I can only touch on this area.

It is worthwhile dealing with effects on physicians as well as on patients and relationships because physicians are people, too, and because what happens to physicians can affect their ability to care for their patients. Thus, L. K. Cartwright (1979), who has discussed sources of distress of persons engaged in health careers, claims there are two major reasons for this study:

> First, to reduce suffering and to restore the capacity to enjoy life to health professionals . . . is a worthwhile goal in its own right. . . . Second, the problems of providers can seriously interfere with the care of patients. . . . the quality of health care will diminish when providers are distressed.

Working with aged patients inevitably brings the doctor into frequent contact with death and dying. There is limited research evidence (e.g., Howard, 1974; Rosenthal et al., 1980) but much opinion that this raises levels of death anxiety among physicians and other clinicians, in some cases to the point of interfering with sound clinical judgment (Linn, Linn, & Gurel, 1973). Support systems or processes can be established in hospital settings to help physicians (Artiss & Levine, 1973) or nurses deal with such anxiety (Vachon, 1979; Vachon, Lyall, & Freeman, 1978). Doctors are probably less vulnerable to such death-related stress than nurses because their contact with the dying is less constant, less of a continuing and personal relationship. However, doctors usually reserve for themselves the burden of conveying bad news of a fatal prognosis, and this is a task not relished (see Rosenthal et al., 1980: Ch. 5).

As noted above, chronic care does not carry the rewards of "saving the patient" (though it has other rewards, such as allowing formation of a relationship with patients who are able more actively and knowledgeably to participate in their own care). Eisdorfer (1973:70) points out that the doctor " . . . is trained not to accept illness but to combat it. . . . the personality of the dedicated individual who will train himself for ten or more years to go into practice is also the kind that would be very frustrated with a situation he sees as hopeless."

Professionals are beginning to attend more carefully to career-related stresses and the possibility of being burned out and becoming listless or apathetic about the results of work and career progress (L. K. Cartwright, 1979; Maslach,1976, 1978). A. Cartwright (1967:172–173), in her study of British physicians in general practice, found highest levels of physician dissatisfaction in doctors who were trained during the 1930s and 1940s. This was a time when medical education was attuned to the hospital, but the National Health Service reorganization changed the focus of general practice away from the hospital in Great Britain. However, as A. Cartwright notes, an alternative to this "inappropriate socialization" kind of explanation is that doctors trained during that period were, at the time of her survey, at a stage in life when they were beset with family and financial worries, one potential source of unhappiness. "It is doctors in this age range . . . who are likely to be most conscious of the present lack of any career structure in general practice."

Gerontologists, in particular, should pay attention to the mutual influence of period, cohort, and aging effects, as these affect the motivation of the physician in care of the aged. Research is needed on burnout in relation to acute and chronic care and in relation to different patient care settings such as solo practice, hospital, and clinic care.

Feelings of being burned out may well interact with the last major aspect of the doctor-patient relationship to be discussed in this review. A lowered morale or optimism concerning one's ability actually to do something useful to help the patient may be associated with a decline in therapeutic activism.

Therapeutic Activism

Physicians vary greatly, both within and between specialty groups, concerning the appropriateness of active and aggressive intervention. For example, some surgeons think others too reluctant to "cut," whereas other surgeons are viewed by their peers in surgery, and perhaps more especially elsewhere, as somewhat too ready to operate. Medical care can vary in its intensity, and some physicians may be more willing than others to rely on natural healing processes, or to use medication, or to give palliative care rather than to seek cure. Therapeutic activism refers to this dimension of the extent to which a physician will actively intervene in pursuit of cure. Therapeutic activism is not invariably better than relative inactivity. However, it is frequently pointed out that, in the case of older patients, there may be an undue tendency toward therapeutic inactivity (see, for example, Breytspraak, 1979; Eisdorfer, 1973; Kart, Metress, & Metress, 1978, Ch. 2). Among the reasons for this are: the belief that impairments and complaints are to be expected in old people, a related failure to diagnose accurately the cause of the complaint, age-related increases in operative risk, an assessment of the merits of active intervention in cost-effective terms (why operate on someone who is going to die soon anyway?), assessment of the merits of intervention in comparison to other alternatives (why resuscitate this patient so she can die next month of cancer?), and, not least, assent to the wishes of patients who may also share this belief that aches and pains and incapacities are to be expected in old age.

Miller and associates (1976) found that twice as many physicians stressed survival of their patients under age 50 than of those aged 75 or more. Of these physicians, however, 38 percent said they put forth equal effort regardless of the age of their patient.

Haney (1971) describes an intervention-maintenance continuum, and argues that "the interventionist is more likely to be disease oriented, whereas the physician characterized by a tendency toward maintenance is more likely to be patient oriented" (Haney, 1971:419). He views specialities such as surgery and neurology as oriented toward intervention; pathology and psychiatry are classical cases of the maintenance modality. These two cases fall at opposite extremes on another dimension: the extent to which the physician is active and the patient passive, on the high-authority pole, represented by pathology, contrasted with mutual participation of physician and patient, as in psychiatric care. Pathology and psychiatry are also at opposite poles of the scientism-humanism dimension in Haney's three-dimensional model. This suggests the independence of the three dimensions. In terms of the analysis I am developing, it implies that therapeutic activism is not inextricably or unavoidably intertwined with authority relationshps or the sureness of epistemological status of the knowledge base.

Diana Crane has described "The Active Physician" in her book on the care of critically ill patients (1975, Ch. 7). Her definition is narrower than my conception of therapeutic activism, in focusing on heroic measures with the critically ill.

Data were gathered from over 3,000 physicians by questionnaire. Using hypothetical cases, Crane developed scales to measure tendencies on the part of the physicians to be active in various dimensions: initiation of resuscitation, performance of heroic operations, and use of heroic treatments (Crane, 1975:26). The most important factor affecting a physician's decision to treat patients actively is the judgment he or she makes of the patient's capacity to perform social roles (Crane, 1975:35, 58–61; see also Brown & Donovan, 1979; Sudnow, 1967:100–116). This social capacity is judged to diminish in older patients, especially in those over age 80.

Activism is also influenced by certain physician characteristics. Liberal Protestants were the least active religious group among internists, and Jews the most active on issues such as resuscitation and use of heavy narcotics dosages for terminally ill patients in pain (Crane, 1975:174–175). The effects of religious affiliation were independent of measures of religiosity, suggesting that a cultural loading on such issues is attained early and persists despite possible biographical changes in religious devotion (Crane, 1975:178; however, Brown & Donovan, 1979, report no religious differences in their study).

It is important to note that Crane found different patterns of religiosity and activism in pediatricians than in internists. Her findings can only be suggestive; and it would be worthwhile obtaining similar data on activism, in Crane's limited sense and in the broader sense I have suggested, from physicians who customarily work with older acute and chronic patients.

Despite a small proportion of lower-class-origin doctors, Crane found that: "There was some indication in the sample of internists that physicians from lower-class origins were more likely to treat patients actively than other physicians. This inverse relationship between social class and activity was also noticeable among the pediatric residents and the surgical samples" (Crane, 1975:173). There was also a slight tendency for men to be more active in their treatment orientation than women (Crane, 1975:173).

A dramatic indication that activism varies according to factors other than the patient's actual condition is reported by Crane (1975:81) with respect to resuscitation procedures in a university hospital. There were fewer resuscitations in May and June than in the other months of the year, and this is attributed to a decline in resuscitations conducted for practice in the technique. This is a setting factor that would not be operative in nonteaching hospitals; it is also, presumably, a factor located in the physician and theoretically measurable by the physicians' desire for knowledge and similar variables.

Therapeutic activism may be related to the affective aspects of the patient physician relationship discussed earlier. Chronic illness seems to lack the drama, and to be devoid of the rewards of effecting cure. "Medical Center" and "Ben Casey" and similar television melodramas seldom deal with chronic care, which lacks the pizzaz of acute care.

Ford (1968) identified several groups of doctors likely to have older patients in their practice. Fifty-eight percent of these doctors did not exhibit any difference in their claimed preferences for patients of any age group. Internists, at 30 percent, were most likely to claim to prefer having elderly patients in their practice, and surgeons, at 18 percent, were least likely to prefer older patients. This is in accord with the interventionist stance of surgeons noted in our discusson of therapeutic activism. The difference between internists and surgeons became even more pronounced when considering chronic patients.

Crane found that physicians in internal medicine distinguish between acute and chronic illnesses and between mental and physical effects of illness when making judgments of activism. However, some physicians did not make these distinctions. Younger physicians appear more likely to make them, and this, Crane suggests, is because they have more direct work experience with such patients (Crane, 1975:63–64).

Therapeutic activism is related to the attribution of a presenting symptom to either disease or aging (see Kart's chapter in this book), and this in turn depends on the knowledge base of the physician. In the relative absence of geriatric training in medical education (Breytspraak, 1978, 1979), it is hardly surprising that physicians and patients share the mistaken belief that many aches and pains are "what you should expect at your age." Coe and Brehm (1973) presented a list of 15 conditions of aging to over 1,500 general practitioners and internists, and asked them to indicate which were thought to be normal conditions of the aging process and which were the result of disease. Many conditions that were in fact disease related were mistakenly considered to be normal aspects of aging. For example, only 42 percent correctly identified senility as disease related, and only 48 percent correctly identified cerebral arteriosclerosis and retinal arteriosclerosis as disease related.

For aged (and also younger) patients, doctors who correctly identified disease-related conditions gave better preventive care as measured by mean number of routine tests and procedures administered to patients. Moreover, older general practitioners performed worse than younger specialists. It was the older general practitioner who was most likely to call a disease-related condition normal. Younger specialists, on the other hand, were more likely to call a normal condition disease related. These findings appear to be consistent with those of Crane on the distinction between acute and chronic, mental and physical illnesses. The explanation for this pattern is not clear.

Therapeutic activism is clearly contraindicated in some cases, and few would favor the unnecessary prolongation of life for its own sake, or for instrumental reasons such as to provide teaching situations for residents or medical students. Many patients clearly do not want to live forever (see evidence reviewed in Marshall, 1980:Ch.6). However, I have suggested that therapeutic inactivity is a problem of special relevance to older patients. Therapeutic activism is one attitudinal domain that is of importance to the doctor-patient relationship because it is directly related to what, in a technical sense, the doctor does to and with the patient.

Interrelations and Implications

Authority is the key dimension of the doctor-patient relationship. This can be seen by imagining that the physician were completely subject to the authority of the patient, dependent upon the patient as a Renaissance painter might depend on a patron in a very different kind of professional-client relationship. Were the physician subject to the authority of the patient, it would matter little whether or not the physician preferred to care for older or younger patients, preferred to be therapeutically active or inactive, or succeeded in persuading the patient to comply with medical advice. It would not matter, that is, to the patient. Giving health care is not, however, like painting a picture.

Despite the tenuous interactional links between patient and physician, their relationship can assume great importance because it ultimately concerns matters of life and death for the patient. Disease almost always has a large socioemotional component, and in the highly charged relationship between patient and physician, the scope of the relationship goes well beyond the technical application of medicine to effect cure of a disease. Not only is the nature of authority different when considering biomedical and psychosocial aspects of the relationship, but, I suggest, authority in the biomedical sphere is in some measure contingent on the nature of the social relationship.

The authority of the doctor continues to be based primarily and fundamentally on expertise. As Antonovsky (1979:202) points out, " . . . the fact that a person has entered the interaction means that he or she has acknowledged that the doctor has a particular competence in dealing with certain kinds of problems—a competence that the patient does not have. . . . The doctor always assumes a relatively superior professional competence." Even technical biomedical authority is far from unbounded, however, as is seen in the case of noncompliance.

To the extent that we can generalize to the broader authority relationship from data concerning compliance or adherence, the greater the ability of the doctor to convey a personalized sense of interest in the patient through high levels of communicative interaction and explanation and through respect for the patient, the stronger is his or her expert authority in that relationship. The authority of expertise or the bureaucratic authority of the office appears to be secondary to and contingent upon the authority of personalized respect. (A better term is needed for this concept, but in effect, it appears that the patient is saying, "if you want me to take seriously your expert advice, you had better treat me as a person and give me a little respect.")

I have tried to distinguish this concern from a concern for highly comprehensive psychosocial care. I do not interpret the evidence as strongly supportive of broad-based psychosocial care. Rather, patients often react to psychosocial care as an unwarranted intrusion on areas of life that they feel that they can take charge of themselves. Antonovsky (1979:206) emphasizes that the authority of expertise is acknowledged by the very fact that the person has gone to see the doctor, placing the patient in a dependent position. A broadening of the scope of that interaction into ever-larger areas of the total person only expands the degree of dependency.

The link between the authority and the affective bonds in the doctor-patient relationship rests on the importance of personalized respect, which is undoubtedly easier to give if the doctor actually likes older patients and their care.

There is a general tendency for many physicians, if not to dislike the aged, to find caring for them unrewarding and less preferred to care of the young. To say this is not to indict doctors because these preferences largely reflect the fact that doctors share in widely held ageist stereotypes. Organized medicine should not be entirely off the hook, however, because the scientism and technological domination of contemporary medicine exacerbates this situation. One physician characteristic that does influence the affective dimensions of the doctor-patient relationship is, therefore, the doctor's stance toward medicine as a science of curing diseases or of healing patients (Antonovsky, 1979:204–206; Engel, 1977b; Haney, 1971).

The overwhelming thrust of contemporary scientific medicine stresses the goal of cure. No wonder, then, that caring for aging and, often, dying patients at times provides little in the way of reward to those who subscribe to the ethos of high-technology medicine. Just as authority is best viewed in processual terms, as negotiated between patients and physicians, the affective qualities of the doctor-patient relationship are ideally seen as unfolding processually over the course of time.

Therapeutic activism is an attitudinal domain of quite direct consequence for older patients. Work experience probably does have a somewhat greater influence with respect to therapeutic activism, because age differences of the doctor on that dimension have been interpreted as indexing differences in experience with older and chronic patients. There are also differences by specialty on this dimension. These probably reflect the interactions of work experience and selection factors (do therapeutically active medical students become surgeons?). In any case, the scanty literature on therapeutic activism also shows the influence of the wider culture, this being most clearly shown in the continuing effects of religious affiliation, regardless of religiosity or religious devotion, on activism in Crane's research on heroic measures. Behaviorally, therapeutic activism also reflects the negotiation success and bargaining strength of patients who may, on the one hand, beg that something be done or, on the other hand, request "no heroic measures."

If there is a big message in this review, it is that individual characteristics of the doctor are probably not as important as setting or organization of care characteristics. If one thinks of the doctor-patient relationship as resting on a fit between two people and two positions, with the positions being that of doctor and that of patient, then we can ask what makes a good fit of people into those interrelated positions. One classical answer to this queston (which is the question of the fit between person and role) is socialization: we think of people learning to want to act in ways appropriate to the expectations for the position. It appears that socialization has not produced a large number of doctors who meet the expectations of patients, or patients who meet the expectations of doctors. Another answer to the "fit" problem is selection: we have carefully to screen role-incumbents and direct them to positions compatible with their own expectations and desires. The problem with the selection position is that patients often effectively lack choice either of disease type or physician type that will affect their position. Doctors also lack choice, or act as if they are not entirely free. They choose specialities because of career opportunities, and their behavior is organizationally constrained.

The third major way to encourage a fit between people and positions is to change the positions. That is, in effect, what is happening now with the positions in the doctor-patient relationship. The relative authority positions between patient and doctor are under review and negotiation, and are being restructured as part of a dynamic larger than the participants themselves. This dynamic has more to do with the characteristics of our political and economic structures than with the motivations, capacities, or background features of physicians. Nonetheless, the micropolitics of the doctor-patient relationship, and the role of physician characteristics in shaping it, are not to be ignored because the macrodynamics of health service delivery do not exist of their own accord. They are realized, made real and consequential, for real human beings in that relationship.

Notes

1. In a recent and very useful paper, Breytspraak (1979) focuses on the way in which health is defined, the extent to which environmental factors are implicated, and the employment of the health team concept as considered in major models of the doctor-patient relationship with older patients.
2. As Hayes-Bautista (1976) points out, patient-practitioner relationships begin as encounters, but often culminate in relationships. This may be especially so in the care of chronic illness.
3. Ben-Sira (1976) argues that: "As a patient is unable to judge the contribution of the content of the practitioner's activities to the achievement of his goal, he confines his judgment to the mode of their presentation (affective behavior)." Pope (1978) reviews a number of studies showing little patient dissatisfaction with technical aspects of care compared to interpersonal aspects and issues such as cost and accessibility (see also Friedson, 1961:175, 208–209).
4. Control over information, therefore, epitomizes the doctor's expert authority. Direct and mediated (through nurses) information control is analyzed in Rosenthal et al. (1980).
5. A. Cartwright cites Davis and Eichhorn (1963), who suggest that friendship leads to *less* compliance with medical regimens. This finding is exceptional, and calls for a more finely grained characterization of the quality of the affective bonds between physician and patient.
6. As expressed by choice of items such as "In making health decisions, the doctor ought to

take a patient's opinion into account," and "It's all right for people to raise questions with doctors about anything they tell you to do."

7. See Bloom & Summey (1978) and their contribution in this book. The conflict approach is articulated by Bloor and Horobin (1975), Collins (1975), Marshall and Tindale (1978–9), McKinlay (1978), Tindale and Marshall (1979), and Waitzkin and Waterman (1974). The negotiated order approach is variously formulated in Danziger (1978), Eisenthal et al. (1979), Hayes-Bautista (1976, 1978), Lazare et al. (1978), Marshall (1978–9, 1980:Ch.6), and Rosenthal, et al. (1980).

8. The same criticism applies to the developmental psychology of aging. Since we have been gathering systematic data about human development through the life cycle for such a short period of human history, it is quite fallacious to claim that we have discovered any universal patterns of human development.

9. As Kogan (1979) observes, " . . . the overall record is a dreary one as far as establishing an attitude-behavior link for the target class of old people." However, there might be stronger links between attitudes and behavior within supportive institutional environments such as hospitals.

10
Problems of Maintaining a Therapeutic Viewpoint

LAWRENCE BRESLAU, M.D.

The special nature of geriatric patients requires that we view them through special glasses so that their unique characteristics and problems can be understood. In particular, the peremptory impact of illness, physical disabilities, and problems of adapting to these changes make special psychological knowledge imperative to the geriatric primary-care physician.

Our purpose here is to illustrate the way in which psychological understanding and technique can be crucial in the care of certain geriatric patients, particularly in those situations where the doctor-patient relationship has deteriorated and the therapeutic point of view of the health-care team has been lost.

Many geriatric patients suffer from irreversible physical disabilities to which they cannot adjust. Unable to overcome their initial response of being overwhelmed by their disability, they persist over long periods with strenuous complaints as though their problems remained acute, and because of their anxiety they cannot work effectively toward rehabilitation. They consequently see themselves as unrehabilitatable, feel increasingly impaired and helpless, and search for ways to transmit this perception to their families, as a way of seeking aid. Although family members may at first respond energetically, they become discouraged and worn out, eventually feel helpless themselves, and transmit these reactions to the doctor. Doctors themselves may begin with a zealous therapeutic attitude, but once feeling the impact of the transmitted discouragement and hopelessness, find themselves trapped in a situation they dread and do not understand but for which they feel responsible. Thus, the doctor gives up his or her expectation of improvement in the patient. Since this reaction is contradictory to his or her own medical value system, the doctor must find ways of justifying the faltering therapeutic attitude.

Let us review a clinical example: A 72-year-old married woman had been a meticulous housekeeper and a dominant force at home through the years. She developed a mild stroke, which affected her right side but interfered only minimally with function. She began to require added assistance from her husband with the preparation of food and housecleaning and help with shopping and transportation from her daughter. This assistance was offered generously by her family for some time until a subtle change came about. Although they dared not share it with each other, the patient's husband and daughter noted their own growing irritation with the amount of help that was required, and began to feel that the need was exaggerated by the patient. At the same time, the patient's requests for help intensified, and she appeared less able to manage aspects of her life that she had handled easily before. When the patient and family brought these new complaints to the physician, he tried carefully to connect the patient's increasing dependency with new, acute biological developments, but was unable to do so. He referred the patient for reevaluation to a neurologist, psychiatrist, and physical therapist, but these specialists were unable to contribute further understanding. When the patient returned to the doctor with unremitting complaints, and the physician had nothing further to offer, he experienced his own reaction of helplessness and irritation. In order to cope with his feeling of impotence, he redefined the patient's problem, and stated that the patient required a nursing home. Since neither the patient nor the family could accept this alternative, which they viewed as a rejection, the relationship between the doctor and patient ended, and the therapeutic effort reached an impasse.

This common sequence of events is diagrammed in Figure 10–1.

The patient's initial perception of the catastrophic disabling event is that there is no possible way out and no possible rehabilitation. Unless the patient has strong emotional and social resources to bring to bear on the situation, he may hold fast to this frightened impression that there will be no cure. Contrary to what one might expect, this reaction presents itself not as an acute clinical depression but as a behavior and a posture characterized by helplessness, passivity, and self-devaluation. This new attitude serves the purpose of warding off the intense depressive effects and of crystallizing a new regressed way of life and relationship to others.

When trying to communicate these feelings, in a continued attempt to be rid of painful feelings and self-perceptions, the patient resorts to primitive psychological mechanisms directed at expelling recognition of the experience and passing it on to others. Such psychological mechanisms are more complex than mere provocativeness, and are difficult to understand. They are typical of infancy, when feeling and functions are shared by mother and child and can be quickly transferred from child to mother in order to gain relief. This process requires not only that the patient wish to

FIGURE 10–1
Diagram of Steps Leading to Therapeutic Impasse

DISABLING ILLNESS
(stroke used as a model)
↓

MOMENTARY EXPERIENCE OF CATASTROPHE
(not necessarily consciously experienced)
↓

ATTITUDE OF HELPLESSNESS WHICH IS TRANSMITTED TO THE PHYSICIAN
(or health care team)
↓

PHYSICIAN'S REACTION, ATTEMPT TO RELIEVE
HIMSELF, AND THE LOSS OF HIS THERAPEUTIC VIEW

be rid of hopelessness but also that the doctor and other members of the health care team function maternally, feel it is their role to take these feelings on as their own, and do so. Many aged have an uncanny way of perceiving how to bring this transfer of feeling about.

Four Fallacies Used by the Physician
to Cope with Patients' Chronic Illness

Once having experienced the patient's transferred emotions, the doctor feels helpless and quietly resentful. With the help of rationalizations —more or less unwittingly—he or she tries in a fashion parallel to the patient to pass on this painful perspective to other members of the health-care team or back to the family. In an attempt to be rid of such reactions to the patient, the doctor uses the existing patterns of health care—the long-term care system, medical specialization, the doctor's autonomy, and ideas concerning the rational limits of medical efficacy. I call these justifications the *custodial fallacy*, the *specialist fallacy*, the *uncooperative patient fallacy*, and the *family responsibility fallacy*.

The *custodial fallacy* is derived from the fact that many aged patients require multiple services that are fully coordinated and are assumed not to be deliverable at home—thus, the need is perceived for custodial settings such as nursing homes. This program of care, however, is frequently inappropriately recommended as a solution to a therapeutic impasse. It is a fallacy because custodial care is not a viable solution in this instance, and the therapeutic impasse is usually intensified by this step.

The *specialist fallacy* employs the medical system of specialization, which allows the physician to define the area of expertise required by the patient. This system of referral is used inappropriately when it becomes a method of deflecting the patient's illness to another area. The physician may feel relieved to define the patient's problem as outside of his or her own expertise.

The *uncooperative patient fallacy* is based on the idea that the doctor alone determines the terms of the relationship with the patient. This view may be invoked particularly when the patient, in an attempt to restore control over the medical situation, may refuse medicine or otherwise refuse to follow the doctor's regimen. Although the doctor may decide that the patient should see someone else under these circumstances, it is fallacious to invoke seemingly explicit rules of medicine rather than carefully to assess the reasons why the patient's illness has shown itself in this way.

The *family reponsibility fallacy* is based upon the idea that the efficacy of medicine is limited and that at times the doctor's role is to interpret these limitations to the family, who in spite of reality, cling to hopes of magical cure. It is fallacious for the physician to judge the patient to be beyond the help of medicine when, in fact, this judgment is influenced by his or her own distress in dealing with the patient's illness rather than by careful diagnosis.

Ultimately, these attempts on the part of the doctor to be rid of the patient's reactions as they are transmitted do remove the patient to another area, where a similar strained set of relationships may repeat with more desperation; the patient may die or regress to a confused state. Another doctor, another nursing home, or another consultation may bring momentary relief and hope, but are frequently a futile exercise.

Overcoming the Impasse

There are perspectives that may make it possible for the physician to maintain the therapeutic point of view when it is challenged. Let us return to the moment the doctor and/or other members of the health-care team begin to feel enveloped by the patient's transmitted helplessness, first feel discouraged and frustrated, and begin to sense a personal need to be free of the patient's problems. Instead of reacting to personal discomfort, the physician must be ready to consider *his or her own reactions* as part and parcel of the *patient's illness* in the same way that he or she may pick up other clinical messages by cues such as the smell of the patient's room or other data derived from the senses. The doctor must then find a way to make this process known to the patient so that the patient may examine his or her own reasons for this behavior. It is sometimes necessary for the doctor to be explicit about the fact that he or she is upset. When this information is brought without punitive intent, it may be possible for patients to examine what they themselves wanted to be rid of and how this was attempted. Thus, the patients can be directed to look once again at their own loss of hope in themselves, in the rehabilitation process, and in the unsolved experience of catastrophe.

The reasons why this strategy has seemed so unavailable are obvious. Neither the doctor, the nurse, nor other members of the team wish to acknowledge the therapeautic impasse when it occurs and especially dread the sharing of their negative attitudes toward the patient.

I should like to present a more detailed case history of a 69-year-old woman.* Since she was a resident in a home for the aged, the medical care system and the social situation around her were different from those of the patient at home. We observed there, however, the same interactions and therapeutic impasses we have already described. There is an advantage in reporting from this setting since the patient's interactions can be more completely evaluated in the somewhat closed system of the home for the aged. Morever, the presence of many participants in the care system—the social worker, the nurse, the nursing aide, the doctor, and the administrator—as opposed to the solitary physician in the community, tends to disperse the patient's reactions and facilitates our analysis of individual facets of behavior.

The patient was a 69-year-old single, diabetic woman, a double lower-extremity amputee who was admitted to a home for aged, "still in shock" in her words, following a second amputation. She lived at a nearby convalescent home for seven months until, after one preparatory visit to the new institution, she was judged ready for admission. Under circumstances of less severe shock, the goals of the preparation process would have been more ambitious, but since much psychological work seemed required to deal with her depression, it was felt that higher goal setting would be more advantageously done after admission.

During the admission evaluation an incident occurred that seemed insignificant and fragmentary but contained a momentous message. During this only preparation visit, Miss G. needed to use the toilet. Although staff members were aware that, as a double amputee, she would require much help, they nonetheless became overwhelmed by the responses that the ensuing interchange engendered in them. The aide staff summarized it as follows: "Miss G. behaved helplessly, and turned over to the staff all respon-

*This case has been previously described and discussed in: The Faltering Therapeutic Perspective, published in the *Journal of Geriatric Psychiatry*, Vol. 13, No. 9, 1980.

sibility for getting to the toilet. This was communicated silently in her total passivity and her simple statement that she would have to use the
toilet. When we tried transferring her from her wheelchair, she acted as
though she had no concept of how this was done, did not help in the transfer, and actually hindered by refusing to let go of the wheelchair and making the staff feel quite *futile*." The aide staff, although they could not justify it objectively, were sufficiently infuriated to state they did not feel the
patient could be managed successfully in the institution. This episode characterized a repetitive pattern of interchange between Miss G. and the
nursing staff around many aspects of nursing care. The tension was frequently augmented by Miss G.'s accusations that the staff was neglectful
of her, and she frequently devalued their work. For instance, she impe-
riously stated: "Goddamn you, you're supposed to help me. What in the
hell do I pay all this money for. Do I have to do everything for myself without you?" As reported numerous times to our weekly staff conference,
aides felt, in response to Miss G.'s behavior, frustrated, depressed, without hope of maintaining a therapeutic attitude, and trapped in Miss G.'s accusations. They appealed frequently for staff help because they could not
tolerate their own rejection of her.

Miss G.'s unit physician, too, finally succumbed to his distaste, and
resolutely suggested that he refuse to remain her doctor; he noted that
were she in private practice, she would be asked to find care elsewhere.
His distress came about through her impulsive departure from her diabetic diet, resulting in an out-of-control blood sugar and a challenge to his
sense of being able to control the illness. His experience of personal helplessness and consequent resentment seemed to motivate his plan to transfer her out of his care.

Miss G.'s social work contacts were particularly to the point. Her
worker sadly remembered repetitive episodes of deep discouragement of
her therapeutic ambitions and professional commitment. She recognized,
"Miss G. seems to feel better if I acknowledge that I have neglected her,
and yet this gives me an uncomfortable feeling about myself." She noted,
however, that, "When I confronted her with her distorting the truth in
order to make me feel guilty, she got sad." This realization tended to block
further confrontations of this sort. She noted: "She seemed to progress
more when I understood her better. I got discourgaged at times and had
no hope of helping her. Nonetheless, it was my job to continue working
with her. I was angry that the doctor would be discouraged and could reject her by invoking his professional role, but that was not within my own
role. I felt I couldn't do it, yet there was no way to express it." Her super-
visor had advised her to get "more involved," but she confided that she
stayed away from Miss G. when possible. She felt, "Miss G. is trying to get

control over me, and I have the fear of giving in." Miss G. had succeeded in dampening the therapeutic effort of the social worker in addition to the already discouraged aides and physician.

Thus, we recognized a series of crises that identified themselves initially as crises within staff members. These heightened moments came at times when our patient felt sorely threatened by a testing of her self-image. Such challenges came specifically when she was asked to consider training for a prosthesis, using an electrical wheelchair, and applying for welfare support. When these events threatened to bring into focus and consciousness her feelings about herself and the experience of injury, she divested herself of these detested elements by *forcing* members of the therapeutic team around her to adopt them as their own.

The social worker's experience of feeling trapped into seeing herself as neglectful to her patient reflects these efforts, especially the patient's attempt to rid herself of the responsibility for "causing" her diabetic gangrene. The image of the "neglectful self," as she attempted to force it upon the social worker and as the social worker resisted, resonated back and forth between the two individuals. The worker astutely noted that if she (the social worker) accepted the blame, the patient felt comfortable. When she confronted the patient with distortion of truth, she (the patient) felt sad. The worker noted that such interchanges caused her to fear that the patient might be "getting the upper hand" and to feel discouraged about further contacts.

The "bad part" of the patient apparently projected on her doctor was her injured ability to control her appetite. Ultimately, *he* felt helpless and out of control, concerned about criticism from peers, and needed to make plans to withdraw himself as her physician.

Although not fully consistent about it, she projected her self-devaluation onto the aide staff. One may have anticipated this response, insofar as the nursing aide is not only the lowest on the basis of job prestige, but also may bring to the situation an already problematic self-esteem based on socioeconomic, cultural, and racial dimensions. It is, thus, not too far afield to ask questions concerning the interplay between the patient's pathological defense mechanisms and the vulnerabilities health care personnel bring to the treatment situation.

The crucial point, then, is that each staff member, by way of the patient's defense mechanisms, experienced the patient's defects as though they were their own. Their attempts to protect themselves from this painful experience formed the basis of a counterreaction manifested by a broad range of nontherapeutic behavior. Recognition of this lapse in the therapeutic point of view became the starting point of therapeutic intervention. When the doctor, nurse, and social worker became able to clarify their distress and by discussion link it to the precipitating stress in the patient, the managing caseworker was then able to bring both of these elements to the patient to be understood.

The worker's transactions with the patient were then directed toward the fact that sufficient progress had been made so that a move to a less-supervised environment could be considered. In the new location, more independent activity and sophisticated social interchange would be available. The patient reacted, predictably, as though attacked, looking for ways to project the potential injury on those around her. The staff was "bad" for suggesting she move. For her, it would be like being "torn" from her present room as though purposely severed from an essential connection. She returned to exhibiting her stumps to others as she had earlier, eliciting from them an anxiety response, especially from the unprepared.

Elements that seemed to be the products of the joint efforts of group and individual casework were apparent. The reactions of the staff were now more bland and professionally distant, and the patient's worker, too, was able to maintain a more professional and therapeutic point of view. She noted as she reacted this time, "All of the previous events, reactions and counterreactions raced through my mind instantaneously. I felt at home with this familiar material, and began once again to call her attention to the process of how I made her feel and how she made me feel." The patient demonstrated increased awareness of her anxiety, and showed an improved ability to concentrate on both the reality and the intrapsychic issues. Thus, although on the basis of current observations we hesitate to make claims, the shift was evident from the primitive defensive posture directed at involving the staff and visitors to reactions that were manageable in the dyadic setting. It was only then that this patient could pay attention to the focal issues that concerned her disability, her deep sadness about it, and the alternative ways of adapting to it.

One must be careful not to attempt to apply these concepts, however, to all aged. We can hope that these concepts will offer further understanding of some aged who have special difficulty with age-determined disability, who may make up only a small percent of the aged population but a very large percent of our patients, and who need a large percent of the doctor's time and attention.

I should like to call attention to a contrasting view to that presented here, by Stern, Smith, and Frank (1953). The authors present "an outline along which we instruct young physicians and social workers about some of the basic mechanisms which come into play during casework with elderly patients." They state further, "Caseworkers and physicians should be made aware of the fact that in working with old clients a good deal of latent anxiety is apt to be precipitated in the worker and physician. The workers should be instructed about the differences between sympathy (which is most important in this type of work) and identification (which is detrimental)." They thus view the negative reaction as originating in a weakness in the physician. Our view is that strong identification with the patient is universal and that the process that ends with the therapeutic impasse begins with the patient's reactions to a disability, and can be understood best on these terms. The identification becomes a weakness when the physician does not understand his or her identification and does not use it in the therapeutic process.

It is time we developed a systematic approach to the ubiquitous problem of the negative therapeutic relationship in geriatric care. Such an approach must rely heavily on psychological expertise. But since a coherent approach to the patient is needed as part of the delivery of primary care, it cannot be left for referral and the psychiatrist's office. Consequently, the primary-care doctor must be trained to think in a systematic psychological way and not simply pay lip service to the idea that aged patients are emotionally sensitive or other platitudes concerning wholistic care. Specifically, the patient's illness must be seen by the geriatric physician as a condition that is frequently totally enveloping. Each participant on the health-care team must be able to see the connection between his or her own reaction and the patient's illness. In order to approach the negative relationships that obtain, a systematic management plan must be formulated through which the aged patient may recognize the way in which distress is dissipated in order to avoid the full impact of the disability. This recognition may help the patient focus on the pertinent issues, work toward adaptation, and allow the health-care team to regain its lost therapeutic perspective.

These remarks characterizing the physician's distress and stumbling way of managing it may seem critical, but they are not intended to be harsh. I hope that what I have suggested can be welcomed by the lonely physician, nurse, or social worker who struggles with the seemingly insoluble personal dilemmas that disabled aged patients unwittingly engender.

PART V
THE CONTEXTS OF CARE

The setting in which elderly patients and physicians meet has significance for the quality of the meeting as well as its outcome. As the contributors to this section make clear, "setting" involves much more than the physical locale of the therapeutic encounter, although that is one issue. The context of care also includes the presence of a health-care team since, often, service is delivered not just by a physician but by an array of providers from different disciplines. On the patient's side, family members, particularly the old person's adult children, are likely to be implicated in relationships with the care providers. Finally, the societal context, the effects of catastrophic events like war and depression, and the varying cultural norms to which older and younger are socialized must be taken into account as well. In terms of Engel's model, the authors in this section concern themselves with most of the top half of the systems hierarchy.

Dr. Estes reviews the issues related to team delivery of care to the elderly, focusing on problems that interfere with team effectiveness. Foremost among these is the inadequacy of financial reimbursement for team members. Nurse practitioners and social workers, two among several critical service participants, are excluded from government payment schemes, partly, Estes proposes, because the caring functions they fulfill are misunderstood and undervalued. One of his solutions is replacement of the fee-for-service system by prepayment methods covering all necessary services. A major organizational problem is the physician's lack of knowledge of the roles and possible contributions of other disciplines, a fact that interrelates with the financial uncertainties to account for the paucity of formal team development in many institutions. Finally Estes is concerned with ways in which teams that do exist fail to confront the need for health system changes, in order best to serve the elderly. As an example, he notes hospital rules and practices that are particularly threatening to aged patients, the lack of rehabilitation services, and inattention to the patient's family network.

One segment of such a network, the old person's adult child, is Dr. Rosow's topic, as he explores the intergenerational ramifications of the family context. Two major sources of disjuncture between generations are the decline of ethnic identity and the rise of educational achievement in the transitional cohort, of which the adult child of the aged patient is likely to be a member. Patient and grown child are from different worlds in their understanding of technology, bureaucracy, and, often, language. Ideally, and perhaps most commonly, the child acts as interpreter, provider of data, negotiator of services, and emotional supporter for the parent. However, the triad of doctor, patient, and child can decay into a two-against-one situation. If the physician is inattentive, tuned out, or has lost his or her therapeutic viewpoint (in Breslau's terms), child and patient may form a coalition to try to force adequate concern and care. Or if the physician is a therapeutic activist (Marshall's term) old person and adult child may coalesce to protect themselves from the physician's zealous attempts to control. Another common two-against-one grouping occurs when doctor and adult child combine, ignoring the wishes of the patient. The likely greater education of the adult child presses for such a combination. Less common is the situation of doctor and patient versus child. Dr. Rosow urges recognition of the various alliances and their meanings as a guide to understanding doctor-elderly patient interaction since it so often involves not two but three interested parties.

The physical settings in which these encounters take place is Dr. Goss' subject. She concentrates on office, hospital, and nursing home, and points out that the patient's own home, an increasingly rare setting for care, is omitted, as are psychiatric and other long-term care hospitals. A deceptively simple but significant difference between doctor's office or clinic and hospital or nursing home is that in the former, the patient goes *to* the practitioner, while in the latter the patient has visits *from* the practitioner. Thus, in offices or clinics, it is the recipient of services who initiates and maintains contact, giving a measure of control to the patient, who, at least in some instances, can go elsewhere if dissatisfied. In hospital or nursing home, however, control lies with the care giver and the institution, and is out of the patient's hands. Differences between settings also occur with respect to the quality of care received, a difficult characteristic to measure. Whether assessed in terms of process or outcome, data on quality by setting are sparse and usually not differentiated by age of the patient. What few data are available, particularly with respect to patient satisfaction, are reviewed.

In the final chapter in this section, Dr. Bloom elaborates on a number of issues at a societal level. Among the contexts of care for those he terms in "advanced adulthood" is the fact that their life experiences have been different from those of younger adults. Echoing Rosow, Bloom reminds us of cohort effects arising from the elderly's experiences of World War I, immigration, and depression. Reviewing the impact of varying socialization practices, he notes the ambiguity of the elderly role, for which no socialization occurs.

The home as a setting for care and for doctor-patient interaction is one area still poorly researched. In view of the U.S. General Accounting Office findings of a few years ago (USGAO, 1979) that much care for the elderly occurs in a family context within the home, this is indeed a lack. Perhaps one justification for its omission as a topic for elaboration in each of the chapters in this section, although it is alluded to in several, is the fact that the thrust of this book is on factors in doctor-elderly patient relationships. Since so few of these now occur in the home, less than 4 percent for those 65 and over according to Goss, inattention to this setting is unfortunately understandable.

11
The Team Context

E. HARVEY ESTES, Jr., M.D.

This chapter assumes that the reader is familiar with the concept of a health-care team in the care of the elderly and accepts that concept. However, it is necessary to specify a few basic points. A team may be large or small, formal or informal, specifically trained or not. A definition by Eaton and Scherger (1978) is helpful: " . . . in organizational terms, a team is a human system which has interdependence in working towards a common goal as its cardinal characteristic." *Human system, interdependence,* and *common goals* are the key words.

We should recognize that this definition permits the inclusion of the patient and the family as members of the geriatric team. Indeed, they are the most important members of the team.

The list of the formally trained professionals who might be included on such a team is almost infinite, but it would certainly include physicians, nurses, physician's assistants, geriatric nurse practitioners, social workers, physical therapists, occupational therapists, speech therapists, dietitians, pharmacists, and administrators. Most teams include a central group of two or three professionals, such as a physician, nurse, and social worker, with others being called in as needed for specific patients with specific problems.

Perhaps the best examples of well-developed geriatric health-care teams can be found in Western Europe, where the presence of centralized health-care systems and funding has encouraged their development. The prototype is the British team, in which the geriatric consultant, the nurse, the physical therapist, the occupational therapist, and the health visitor meet regularly to solve patient care problems arising in a defined area. In this setting, the consultant also has a set of special-purpose facilities at his disposal, consisting of an acute-assessment ward in a general medical/surgical hospital, a rehabilitation unit, and a variety of long-stay nursing units. The system also provides home care services and other supports, which can be deployed as needed by a given patient.

When such health-care teams exist, there is no doubt that they are highly effective. The problems of inadequate physician time and poor access can be solved. Services of high quality can be provided at a reasonable cost. Patient acceptance of such teams has been uniformly high. The only difficulty with acceptance in most settings in this country has been in the professional area, particularly among physicians. Professionals working in such teams recognize their advantages to both patients and team members. Interprofessional support, so important for high-quality care, can be achieved in such an arrangement.

In spite of these advantages, very few such organized systems exist in the United States. It is much more typical that *no* organized system exists. An acute medical or surgical problem is managed by a physician in a hospital setting, and at the very end of the patient's stay, the social work service is asked to place the patient in a suitable long-stay unit, or to arrange for visiting nursing services. Prior to this point, there has been no interaction between professionals, and certainly no discussion about what is best for the patient. It is no wonder that in most cases the nursing home becomes the recourse of least resistance and the "solution" for many patients, whether it is appropriate or not.

The past decade has brought a rapid increase in the number of primary-care clinics and in the number of training programs for family physicians and primary-care internists. These programs have recognized the many advantages of effective health-care teams; federal grants have included inducements for the formation of such teams and explicitly for the inclusion of nurse practitioners.

In spite of all of these advantages to both patients and professionals and in spite of the inducements offered through federal funding, most objective observers would concede that there has been very slow movement toward formally organized teams, either in the health-care field as a whole, or in geriatric care. The team concept has had little impact on the main stream of medical care. Health-care teams formed under federal grants have a high mortality rate after the grants expire. Most of the teams that do exist are under institutional rather than medical-practice sponsorship.

Rather than elaborating on the advantages of such teams, the remainder of this chapter will analyze the reasons that have discouraged their formation and in some instances caused their demise. These factors must be understood and addressed if these highly productive units are to succeed.

In this conception, there are environmental problems, there are organizational problems, and there are functional problems. The first type are the most difficult because they are embedded in a larger societal framework and are not directly under professional control.

Environmental Problems

The environmental problems relate to payment for the services provided by such teams. The ideal base for the operation of geriatric teams is a primary-care clinic or a private-practice setting. Part B of the Medicare law limits payment to those services that are directly provided by the physician, plus those services, such as injections and dressing changes, that are directly ordered by the physician. The regulations specifically prohibit payment for those activities that might be most useful in a geriatric-care team.

In many states, these regulations are widely ignored, but when invoked, the restrictions are apt to cause particular problems for teams trying to expand their functions in creative ways. This erratic use of regulations is apt to discourage the formation of health-care teams in the private-practice settings. Exceptions have been made for rural health clinics, but the required modifications of the accounting system and the reporting requirements are so cumbersome and tedious that pursuit of this exception is discouraged.

There is another, and even more fundamental, problem with the payment system. Our payment system is a fee-for-service system on which has been superimposed an insurance system. For proper operation of such a system, there must be a well-defined unit of service upon which payment is based. A day of hospitalization, an appendectomy, and a radiologic film of the chest are examples of well-defined units of service that are the same, or approximately so, wherever performed. The more vague and general the service, the more difficult it becomes to assign it a monetary value. Under such a system, the most important function, the caring function, carries no value, because it cannot be defined.

The result of this system is that the primary-care components in the medical-care system have been tremendously undervalued. The only unit of reimbursement in most ambulatory settings has been the office visit, and the insurance systems, for their own protection, have placed a very low value on such visits. All primary-care functions suffer under such a system, and, as a result, a preponderance of funds flows into specialty and subspecialty care of a technical variety. Such a financial disadvantage threatens training and the total viability of primary care of all kinds, whether geriatric, pediatric, internal medicine, or whatever.

My opinion is that primary-care services, including the services of health-care teams, should be paid for through a prepayment or capitation system. Secondary and tertiary care could continue to be paid on a fee-for-service basis, but I think that the primary-care physician or team should be the gatekeeper for these services.

Organizational Problems

Another basic problem that plagues our geriatric-health-care teams is that there are discontinuities between professional members of most such teams. Each professional tends to be very well trained in his or her own field, but does not have the breadth of experience or training to acquaint him or her with the functions of the others on the team. This is especially true in the case of the physician, who is most often called upon by tradition and by legal requirements to lead the team. For optimal functioning, the physician and all other team members must be able, either by experience or formal training, to do most of the common tasks of all others. Only in this way can each appreciate the techniques and the problems of the other members.

Another organizational problem is that there has been little formal health-team development activity in most geriatric settings. Out of experience in neighborhood health centers and other primary-care sites in the late 1960s and early 1970s grew a body of knowledge and specific designs for team development activities. Among these designs is that of Dr. Irwin Rubin and colleagues (Rubin, Plovnick, & Fry, 1975), who proposed a self-instructional format of seven educational modules. This series is completed by the entire working team, a process requiring about 21 hours. The result of such activity is the explicit designation of goals, roles, relationships, leadership, and communication formats. In spite of the existence of such strategies and a considerable body of evidence attesting to their effectiveness in developing a true team, they have seldom been employed in practice settings.

These last two problems are organizational problems that are within the control of the professionals involved in the formation and operation of health care teams. Why have they not been solved? In my opinion, it is related to their high cost in time, energy, and dollars.

In this way, these two problems are interrelated with the payment problem. The lack of a payment system that will support a geriatric team creates a situation in which there are few incentives for those interested in such a system to invest their time and energies to achieve cross-disciplinary training and formal training in team interaction.

Functional Problems

A common functional failing of geriatric teams is their failure to work for needed modifications of the setting of patient care. Attention is confined to the patient and his or her problem, without recognizing that system changes are necessary for maximum benefits. The major problem in most areas is the hospital. Almost every aspect of the hospital environment is a threat to the elderly patient. The physician orders medications and interventions as though the patient had the same homeostatic reserves and the same excretory and metabolic capacity as the younger patient. Nurses take away shoes and clothing and enforce bed confinement. Routines and preferences are violated, ad infinitum.

Ideally, each acute medical and surgical hospital should have a ward setting in which the entire staff is attuned to the elderly patient and to which all such patients are admitted. A given doctor might still be unaware of the differences between young and old, but a good staff of nurses and consultants would go a long way in acting as advocates for the patient should one such staff member fail in his or her functions.

The geriatric team should work toward the establishment of geriatric assessment wards and rehabilitation units, which would enhance and extend the team's services to more patients. Such a setting would enable them to teach, by example, their skills to other professionals in the community.

Another functional failure of many geriatric-health-care teams is their lack of attention to the patient in his or her home setting and to the network of family and friends of which the patient is a part. These problems and a number of others remain to be addressed by geriatric-health-care teams.

Summary

This chapter has attemped to analyze those factors that have prevented the widespread adoption of a highly acceptable and effective system for providing health care to the elderly. Environmental problems, organizational problems, and functional problems all contribute to the failure of this system to thrive. In this connection, it is well to remember the hierarchical system in Engel's conception (Chapter 1). The environmental problems of payment systems exist at a very high level of complexity—the level of the society and the nation. The organizational problems related to the training and experience of teams exist at the level of the community. The specific functional shortcomings of teams in addressing improved institutional settings of care, home environment, and family also involve the community and family levels of the hierarchy.

It should be pointed out that the individual health-care professional has less and less *direct* control over interactions as the focus moves up the hierarchical levels of organization. Thus, the most difficult of these problems to correct will be that at the highest level—the payment problem. The only answer is to begin to recognize these problems and to make others aware of them so that we can act in concert to correct them.

12
Coalitions in Geriatric Medicine

IRVING ROSOW, Ph.D.

As enlightened gerontologists are aware, the field of gerontology is changing. It has entered a transition because the nature of older people is undergoing change. The newly emerging young-old and their slightly younger siblings differ in significant ways from the old who went before. This new cohort—the men and women now roughly between 55 and 70 years of age—represents a generation of transformation. They reflect some fundamental social changes that distinguish them from their predecessors and may even prefigure a new gerontological rhetoric.

How do the generations differ most significantly? For our purposes, two related characteristics sharply discriminate the past old from the future old—or in a figurative sense, our transitional generation from their parents. These cardinal features are the decline of ethnicity and the rise of education. The very old are more ethnic and less educated than their children.

The Decline of Ethnicity

The present group of the old-old, those over 75, includes the last survivors of the massive waves of immigration before the first World War and some of the lesser wave of refugees from Nazi Germany during the 1930s. This is the generation of immigrants whose life was rooted in the ethnic community and ethnic institutions. Not only were there local churches, mutual aid societies, fraternal orders, businesses, banks, and foreign language newspapers, but also there were the informal systems that welded them into a viable community. These local organizations did not preclude immigrants' assimilation to the United States; indeed, they fostered Americanization. But this was anchored in a strong ethnic tradition that kept people's identity bicultural. Accordingly, they considered themselves and were regarded by others as hyphenated: Polish-Americans, Swedish-Americans, Anglo-Americans. Some of them were so embedded in the ethnic community that they scarcely learned English, but they were the exceptions.

The point, however, is not how encapsulated was their ethnic existence, but rather its vibrance and centrality in their lives. It remained viable for them not only during the first half of this century, but also later in the face of many profound social changes, including for many, their own eventual prosperity and their creation of new ethnic settlements in the suburbs, watered down, cleaned up, and modernized perhaps, but clearly visible and still viable for them. Out of the ghetto, they became successful ethnics, but they were still ethnics.

For their children, however, the middle-aged adults of our transitional generation, ethnicity has declined as a vital force. America has not become the ultimate melting pot whose vision quickened the pulse of sociologists and other savants 50 years ago—in this they were wrong. But if ethnicity has not disappeared, neither has it flourished and retained strength as a critical force in social organization (except in a narrow sense where local minorities have held the balance of political power). In a pluralistic society, ethnicity has lost its structural importance in contrast to factors such as race, social class, and economic institutions. Other memberships and associations are more powerful.

So ethnicity is alive, but not vigorous. It has lost much distinctive earthiness and bite, become more formalized, self-conscious, and superficial. The vitality that once sprang unbidden from the loins of life—the common daily round, mutual dependence and aid, a shared status, and similar fate—now must be deliberately sought, stimulated, and cultivated, much as one must nurture a sickly child.

Nowhere is the evidence of these changes so clear as in the fate of mother tongues. They still survive in encapsulated communities. But among assimilated ethnic groups, which are in the majority, mother tongues have virtually expired. When I was growing up in the 1930s, Yiddish was universally spoken and read by immigrants of my parents' generation. But among their children, my transitional generation, the figure is substantially less than 10 percent, and among our children, only a fraction of 1 percent. This is an attrition rate of more than 90 percent with each successive assimilated generation. Similarly, during the 1930s, at least half a dozen national newspapers were published in Yiddish. They thrived, for they represented the vital interests of their people, including special constituencies within the Jewish community. The market support was there, and you could pick up any of them at any drugstore, candy store, or grocery in a Jewish neighborhood. By now, most of them, including several of the largest, have perished. Only one is carried (in a downtown shop) even by San Francisco's most comprehensive newspaper dealer. What is most impressive is the difficulty of learning the fate of these papers from journalistic reference books and journalists, including those publishing the local English-language Jewish week-lies. Nobody knows anything about papers and publishers that once were bywords of Jewish life across the country.

The fate of the Yiddish national press epitomizes the fate of most ethnic journalism. With assimilation and the decline of the native language, the distinctive set of ethnic interests, material and cultural, shrinks. So the market for an ethnic press may or may not come to approximate zero, but it is certainly uneconomic, and can no longer sustain publication. This simply expresses the decline of ethnicity between the immigrants and their children, the transitional generation.

The Rise of Education

In the last fifty years, waning ethnicity has been paralleled by a steady increase in public education. With the growing complexity of our economy and other institutions, the level of public education has risen drastically.

For our purposes, this development has two key features. First, after World War II, education expanded dramatically. Pressures for more schooling were exerted everywhere, increasing the years of education in all social classes. The GI Bill particularly introduced a revolutionary concept: higher education on a wholesale scale. In a sharp departure from elitism, this popularized the university and opened its gates to vast segments of youth who otherwise would never have seen a quadrangle. Once launched, the public financing of education for many was continued in numerous forms: benefits for military service, support of selected professional and other programs, and various other public subsidies of education.

Secondly, the first beneficiary of this educational growth was our transitional generation, those now about 50–70 years of age. These are mainly veterans of World War II and the Korean War, who in the late 1940s and 1950s, flooded the campuses for a college education. They represent the greatest educational watershed in history, sharply demarcating themselves from those who passed before. Nowhere is the educational difference between successive cohorts greater than that between the immigrant and the transitional generations.

In the first three decades of this century, immigration indexed not only ethnicity, but extremely limited education. The following analysis is predicated on major educational differences between generations. Thus, although immigrants are the extreme case, the general analysis actually goes far beyond them to embrace all poorly educated aged with well-educated children.

The Family Context

Though we have spoken here only in demographic terms, the forces at work in the larger society also played themselves out in the immigrant family. We must make no mistake: education and the social mobility it engendered were powerful forces of assimilation that profoundly changed the experience and lives of the transitional generation from those of their immigrant parents, whatever their love for each other. With the best will in the world, a retired farmer could absorb just so much Boolean algebra or corporate tax law and his widowed sister just so much Sigmund Freud or Benjamin Spock. Similar problems obtained outside the spheres of work and science, indicating the extent to which the two generations lived in different worlds that overlapped mainly in their family ties.

For our purposes, the crucial differences center on their modes of thought, their relations to the worlds of science, technology, and bureaucracy in their modern institutional contexts. This made for great differences in the generations' sophistication, adaptablilty, and comfort in dealing with professional settings and services. Such basic differences would only be amplified in the older generation by any impediments of language, competence, or dependence that would limit their ability to deal with medical personnel and situations.

The quality of these differences is certainly more important than their extent. Members of the transitional generation are more familiar and comfortable with the world of modern medicine than their uneducated parents, and they deal with it much more capably, even fluently. This is the basis on which adult children become active parties in their parents' health care—specifically, "taking mama or papa to the doctor." The children communicate effectively with the medical establishment, so they are involved in almost all care, from checking out some chronic constipation to heading for major surgery. The adult child acts as an agent, mediating between an old parent and the doctor. This intercession does not necessarily commence in old age, for its foundation is usually laid earlier. But it assumes increasing importance in later life as the decline in an old person's health requires greater medical attention.

The Model Case

Under ideal conditions, the child's mediation should work out very well, for he or she serves as an interpreter in several necessary ways:

1. Language (the medium): if there is any linguistic barrier between

doctor and patient, the child can usually bridge the gap in both directions.
2. Objectivity (the facts): the child facilitates the exchange of necessary information back and forth.
3. Interpretation (the meaning): the child conveys explanation, sets facts in perspective and clarifies their meaning for both parties.

Beyond this neutral facilitation, the child also takes on two more active functions.

4. Negotiation: the child usually enters actively into the decision about treatment, the choice of what should be done and how. This direct participation may vary from persuasion through buffering to exerting pressure. Such activity is only to be expected, for a child is not simply a catalyst, but a party with vital interests in the proceedings.
5. Emotional Support: the child also normally provides a parent with emotional support in facing the medical situation—the problem, the treatment, the consequences, and their implications.

This model case is ideal, and it is essentially rational. It is based on the sensible premise that helping the older patient is the sole consideration for everybody and that all efforts are bent to this purpose. Such goodwill and a common goal do not always spread sweetness and light, but they should at least assure enterprise and cooperation in helping the old patient. This is mainly the case, this is how it usually works—but not always. And it is the exceptions, the troublesome cases, that concern us here.

The Uncertain Triad

Social scientists are pleased when the virtue of ideal models is served, but experience has made them cautious. Nagging questions persist about whether children's intercession is always what it seems to be and whether it is really optimal. For doctor, patient, and adult child are three people —to small group researchers, a *triad*. And triads do have some interesting properties. There have always been model triads, harmonious and cohesive, which together have been more than the sum of their parts. Examples include the Three Wise Men, Botticelli's Three Graces, Macbeth's Three Witches, the Three Musketeers and Charlie's Angels, to put them chronologically. So triads are often congenial and coherent.

But not always; they can also be erratic. One of the cardinal results of small group research is that triads may be notoriously unstable, losing their unity and decaying into coalitions of two against one. While not invariant, such cleavage is extremely common. Thus, coalitions are virtually endemic and certainly latent in triads.

So it may be with doctor, older patient, and adult child. Their triadic structure may catalyze possible conflict and alliances which turn two against one and may sacrifice the rational order to other interests. Therefore, let us now look at some of the possible coalitions, both rational and irrational, that arise in geriatric medicine. We will briefly review the three sets of pairs and the odd one out.

Parent + Child vs. Doctor

Perhaps we can start with the clearest, if possibly the most stereotyped group of cases. This includes all variations of the set in which the doctor takes only a perfunctory interest in the older patient. There may be many reasons for this. The doctor may be terribly busy and harassed, some critically ill patient may be on his mind, so the geriatric patient may not have his full attention. Or he may regard geriatric patients in general as "old crocks," beset with various aches, pains, creaks, and complaints, the final effluvia of chronicity. Many of these are not terribly serious or consequential; medically, they are not interesting or stimulating, but only dull, dull, dull. There is really no effective treatment for many of these ailments, only a bit of analgesic relief, so that the doctor can do little to help the body. This is only compounded if the geriatric patient is also a hypochondriac (with or without hysterical overtones) whose imaginary complaint can drive the physician with limited time and energy straight up the wall. Under such circumstances, it is understandable that the doctor's attention, a precious resource, may wander elsewhere.

These cases involve common, routine conditions with a fundamental stamp of inevitability, irreversibility, and "normal" deterioration. To this extent, they are open invitations to inattention, quick pigeonholing and stereotyping, as the dismissive expression "old crock" readily affirms. They resemble other classes of stereotyped patients, including the well-educated woman known in the trade as the "neurotic middle-class housewife."

There are also other consequences of stereotyping. This may result in premature closure that misses or discounts a significant condition. Thereby, examination and tests are limited and the diagnosis compromised. Further, physicians are very familiar with vague, ineffable complaints. Indeed, some symptoms beyond malaise are extremely difficult to describe. But where doctors make allowances for this in younger, especially articulate patients, the stereotyping of the old may convert ineffable condition to vague mentality, leading to ready discount of the symptom. Thus, a burden of proof may be subtly transferred to the geriatric patient.

What these and other stereotyped cases have in common is the frequency with which the doctor may tune out and not listen, substituting the odds of probability for careful diagnosis. For the patient, there is a legitimate problem, but for the physician, there is no condition he can really treat. What registers for the patient and his or her child is their apparent inability to get through to the doctor. This, then, becomes one major basis of the parent-child coalition: to make the doctor hear, to get him to turn on, tune in, and get with it.

In some cases, the doctor may be shedding some of his legitimate responsibilities, wittingly or by default. But other coalitions are directed against just the reverse: the physician's effort to control the patient beyond what is reasonable. The doctor's conception of the good, necessary, and right may infringe on the patient's autonomy and options. In such instances, the patient and child may unite to defend the patient from the doctor's zeal and muscle.

But, as I have indicated, coalitions are not simply directed at the physician's derelictions. Often, the doctor is the reluctant agent of a grim reality that patient and child refuse to accept. In terminal illness, there is nothing the doctor can do to change the outcome. Yet patient and child may unite against the doctor to demand magic, to change or undo that which cannot be changed or undone. Or they may unite in a collusive denial of reality, casting the doctor in the role of a villain who withholds remedy and salvation.

So both sides of the coalition against the professional have grievances, and the sheer fact of an alliance cannot assure us where the virtue lies.

Doctor + Child vs. Parent

Perhaps the most frequent type of doctor-child alliance occurs when these two effectively ignore the patient and deal directly with each other as principals. The child is then no longer strictly an agent or representative. Instead, child and physician enter into direct negotiation about treatment, basically discounting the patient as an interested party. The old parent is presented with the results as a fait accompli.

Sometimes this reflects a genuine incompetence of the patient, one that might literally warrant a power of attorney in legal affairs. If the parent's competence is really questionable, this involves a delicate balance: to locate that point to which the parent's judgment can be trusted, after which the child's judgment should take over. But, usually, competence is not at issue, and cases have been known where the parent's judgment was superior to the child's to the very end.

This pattern is not necessarily malicious, and may even be innocent, for it is predicated on doctor and child acting in good faith in the patient's best interest. Nonetheless, there is a quiet, sometimes unconscious arrogation of the patient's prerogatives that is at best patronizing and at worst deperson-alizing and dismissive of the older person. The parent may seldom be accorded the courtesy of significant choices that are well within his or her competence. With the doctor's cooperation, all this occurs in the name of the child's acceptance of responsibility. Because it is also a very efficient alliance, time pressures on the doctor are also conducive to it.

Whatever the result, this pattern is at least benign in its motives. The best interest of the parent presumably governs the intercession. But this is opposed by another pattern that places the child's concerns first. He or she may want to maintain control of the situation for various reasons: to keep the authority for final decisions, to minimize personal inconvenience, responsibility, demands, or even costs in the treatment and care of the parent. Consequently, the child may exert subtle influences and pressures to assure the decisions he or she wants by alliance with the doctor.

An additional pattern arises when an adult child looks to the doctor for vindication and support of his or her position in a dispute with the parent. The disagreement may legitimately center on the illness, or this may be only a convenient cover for other problems in the relationship. But the support of the physician becomes a prime resource in the dispute and the basis of an alliance.

The crucial factor for the doctor is how similar these patterns may seem, even though they arise for different reasons. He may not only be manipulated for improper purposes, especially by a sophisticated child, but if he is too distracted, trusting, or oblivious the manipulation might even have an adverse effect on the medical decision.

Of course, if the physician is struck by the child's unreasonable pressure or importunity, he may feel that the patient needs some protection and cast his influence on behalf of the parent. So let us now turn to consider this kind of alliance.

Doctor + Parent vs. Child

In general, the coalition of doctor and patient is usually, but not invariably, in the parent's defense. The doctor tries to redress an imbalance of power between parent and child by lending his authority and influence to support the patient. Just as in the parent-child coalition, where the child acts as the parent's agent, so in the parent-doctor alliance does the doctor act as the parent's friend in court. Not quite as a representative, but also more than a silent partner.

Now, what might the physician be defending the parent against? He might be contending with a variety of filial incursions: abrogation of the parent's rights, arbitrary control by the child, arrogation of legitimate parental choices or decisions, blind zeal and overconscientiousness, the shedding of proper filial responsibility, the child's dogmatism and pride. Most of these involve issues of power.

But there are at least two other cases in which the patient needs protection from the adult child. The first is the child's sheer fear of what is happening to the parent. This is no longer a matter of sympathy, but of projection. The child does not react to the illness realistically as a condition of the parent, but as if it were his or her own. Thereby, the child's response is governed by his or her own fear of the perceived threat. Whether the parent might be able to cope with the threat realistically or not, there is the problem of limiting hysteria or contagion, of fixing clearly who is sick and who is not. Sometimes doctor and parent must cooperate to reassure and stabilize the child.

Similarly, there may be the element of a child's guilt. This may develop if he or she regards any deterioration in the patient as a sign of personal failure, a reflection on the child's concern (omnipotence?) in caring for the parent. In such cases, it may take the joint effort of doctor and patient to reassure him or her of the realities and absolve the child of guilt.

Whenever there is a split between parent and child, an endemic problem is that the physician generally casts the deciding vote. This virtually assures that if he is not manipulated outright, at least his support will be wooed. Therefore, he must exercise care in taking sides. His basic problem is how to make the best decisions and recommendations without being forced into an embroiled partisanship.

Conclusion

The examples we have considered are not a simple portrait of heroes and villains, of egoists and victims, but of human beings with normal strengths and frailties caught up in sometimes charged circumstances. They touch on the range and complexity of the problem, although they are by no means complete and certainly are not an analysis. Indeed, for one who is neither a medical gerontologist nor familiar with the territory, a systematic analysis would be presumptuous.

But it is not inappropriate to suggest a conceptual approach to the problem. Much of geriatric medicine takes place in a triad. Not all such relationships are weak or narrow; indeed, most of them are not. But many do become problematic, subject to hidden agendas and instability, and it is these that concern us.

As we have seen, the sheer fact of an alliance is no reliable guide to its significance or to whose interests prevail. Similar structures can serve various purposes. To untangle this problem and its relation to proper medical practice, we might well examine the function of coalitions in dealing with four specific variables:

1. inequalities of power,
2. where control resides,
3. where responsibility is lodged or shed, and
4. whose views of the situation are vindicated.

Conceiving the geriatric professional relationship as a triad certainly facilitates this analysis. Different permutations of these variables should indicate those particular variants of each coalition that tend to be problematic and how they may be recognized. This promises to bring some order and clarity to behavior that otherwise seems only senseless and perplexing. The triad provides a heuristic key to whose interests are being served and what these are. There is a rich literature on coalitions in the triad that can inform this study.

The big waves of immigration are behind us, and the more recent ones are much smaller, but this does not signify that this professional problem will disappear. We may expect that triads in geriatric medicine should continue in the future when families display a sharp increase in the dependency of the old or the education of the young. Both these factors, but especially educational differences, exert strong pressures toward doctor-child coalitions.

13
Situational Effects in Medical Care of the Elderly: Office, Hospital, and Nursing Home

MARY E. W. GOSS, Ph.D.

In 1975, elderly people in the United States made some 141 million visits to physicians, averaging 6.6 visits per person per year (National Center for Health Statistics, 1979). They were patients in short-stay hospitals for a total of 64 million days, with an average length of stay in the hospital of 12 days per person discharged (National Center for Health Statistics, 1977). Close to one million of the elderly resided in nursing homes in 1973–1974, where the median length of stay for all residents—including those under age 65—was 547 days (National Center for Health Statistics, 1977).

This chapter describes some of the ways in which these different contexts of health care—office or clinic, short-term hospital, and nursing home—affect relationships between aged patients and physicians. Analyzed first is a major structural difference among the three settings that has important implications for the social nature of the doctor-patient relationship. Then an overview is presented of what we know and do not know about the quality of medical care in the three settings, in terms of patients' satisfaction with care—the psychosocial dimension—and also in terms of technical medical dimensions.

Before focusing on these topics, however, it is worth calling attention to the fact that this list of settings omits psychiatric hospitals as well as other long-term hospitals, which are too diverse for attention here. The list also omits a context of medical care that was historically important: the patient's home. When Wilson described the different social settings for the doctor-patient relationship in the early 1960s, he reasonably began with the home as a context for care. Only then did he consider, in turn, the practitioner's office and the hospital (Wilson, 1963). Many people are old enough to remember having been visited routinely by their family doctor when sick in childhood; house calls by physicians were quite common in the United States at least until the early 1940s. And as late as 1959, house calls represented almost one-tenth (9.2 percent) of all physician visits (Goldsmith, 1979).

Although the home remains a major setting for medical care in some parts of the world, in the United States interaction between doctor and patient in the patient's home has become statistically rare. In 1971, only 1.7 percent of physician visits were house calls (Goldsmith, 1979). By 1975–1976, the proportion of physician visits represented by house calls had declined further to 1.2 percent. In that period, house calls constituted 3.7 percent of all physician visits for those aged 65 and over, and less than 1 percent for persons under age 65 (calculated from Table 77, pp. 272–273, in National Center for Health Statistics, 1978). Patients' requests for home visits are often met with disbelief, or countered with physician requests to come to the emergency room of the local hospital. And in some cases where home visits are part of the services contracted for, as in some prepaid plans, the home visits may be provided by another set of physicians hired by the plan exclusively for that purpose. In brief, the home is no longer a major setting for physician-patient interaction in the United States, even though a good deal of health care occurs there (Shanas & Maddox, 1976).

Context and Control

Putting aside the home and the long-term hospital, therefore, and considering the three other contexts of interaction, we start with a very simple observation. Office and clinic care involves visits *to* the doctor. Hospital and nursing home care, however, involves visits *from* the doctor.

In the office or clinic situation, therefore, whether or not a doctor-patient relationship even begins depends primarily on the patient, not the doctor; the patient must first arrive at the office or clinic in order for interaction to take place. In the same vein, whether or not a given doctor-patient relationship is maintained over time through office or clinic visits depends largely on the patient, who may choose not to keep appointments regularly, or to sever the relationship entirely and go to another doctor or clinic (if he or she lives in an area where there is a choice, of course, and can afford to make the choice).

What we are talking about here is control over the initial formation and continued existence of the doctor-patient relationship. And in the case of the ambulatory patient who receives care in a doctor's office or clinic, this basic form of control lies largely in the patient's hands rather than the doctor's (Friedson, 1961; Stimson, 1978). This is a potent form of control, obviously, since it means that so long as they are reasonably ambulatory, patients may "shop" for physicians (Kasteler et al., 1976) within the limits of income and available doctors, and may register dissatisfaction simply by not returning to the office or clinic, in other words, by terminating the relationship.

In contrast, once a patient is hospitalized or living in a nursing home, the locus of control over the existence and maintenance of the doctor-patient relationship is likely to shift to the doctor, if only because both of these situations are structured so that it is the doctor who makes the visits, not the patient. Even though the hospital or nursing home patient be ambulatory and not bed-bound, it is the doctor who determines whether—and how often—he or she sees the patient, at what time of the day or night, and how long the encounter will last. In such circumstances, control over maintenance or cessation of the relationship is, in effect, out of the patient's hands, particularly for patients in nursing homes, who are less likely to have relatives ready to besiege the doctor with inquiries and requests that may necessitate an unplanned doctor visit.

Of course, assuming that the hospitalized patient recovers sufficiently to be discharged into the community and becomes an actual or potential office or clinic patient again, he or she may again exert more control over the relationship. But the nursing home patient who remains in the nursing home and never again returns to the status of office or clinic patient never again regains control over the doctor-patient relationship. Except in relatively rare cases, the nursing home patient is a truly captive participant in the relationship or, more often, a passive recipient of medical care.

The extent to which a patient has control *over* the doctor-patient relationship naturally may be expected to affect the extent of a patient's control *in* the relationship. While not denying the relevance of the conceptual models of the doctor-patient relationship that emphasize role asymmetry and the doctor's authority to control patients and events in their lives (Bloom, 1965; Bloom & Summey, 1978; Parsons, 1951; Szasz & Hollender, 1956; Wilson, 1963), Freidson (1961) has pointed out that institutionalized patients are much more subject to physician authority than are office patients. In client-dependent office practices particularly, where the physician relies on his or her patient's good opinion for new referrals, the power of the patients to influence physicians' actions may be considerable (Freidson, 1961; 1970c). For patients in hospitals and especially for patients in nursing homes, however, such power is rare or nonexistent, except perhaps for the very rich.

There are other notable structural characteristics of office, hospital care, and nursing home care—such as variation in the number of doctors and other personnel with whom a patient typically interacts in the three settings—that deserve examination and comparison in terms of their impact on doctor-patient relationships. Rather than pursue this task here, however, attention will be given to a related and perhaps ultimately more important topic: the quality of medical care in the three settings.

Context and Quality

By way of background, it is necessary to note that in the relatively short history of systematic medical care evaluation, three different approaches to the task have evolved. The approaches are usually labeled according to the types of variables examined to determine quality, namely, structural variables, process variables, and outcome variables (Brook & Williams, 1975; Donabedian, 1966; 1977).

Structural variables in medical care consist of the formal qualifications and organization of those who provide care, as well as the characteristics of the setting for care, including physical facilities and equipment. *Process* variables in medical care consist of the behaviors of the practitioner: what the practitioner does to, for, and with patients in the course of caring for them. Process includes clinical history taking, physical examination, ordering tests, making diagnoses, prescribing appropriate therapy and/or preventive measures, performing surgery, communicating, and being supportive. *Outcome* variables refer to the results of care, not to the ways in which the care was given. Two major types of outcome have been of interest in this approach to quality evaluation: clinical (technical/medical) outcomes and psychosocial outcomes. A clinical outcome is the state of health of a patient that results from the care received; a psychosocial outcome is how the patient feels about the care he or she has received, in other words, the extent of satisfaction. The two types of outcome are not interchangeable. Patients have been known to be satisfied with medical care that is technically poor, and technically good care does not necessarily lead to satisfied patients (see, for example, Trussell, Morehead & Ehrlich, 1962).

Satisfaction with Care

While there have been a number of isolated, small-scale studies of patients' satisfaction with their medical care over the years (Lebow, 1974), there have also been occasional surveys using national samples. These nationwide surveys are of special interest here.

Office/Clinic Care. In 1955, before Medicare and Medicaid, the National Opinion Research Center of the University of Chicago (NORC) carried out a sample survey of the U.S. adult noninstitutionalized population to determine, among other things, how satisfied Americans were with the care and treatment they had received from doctors during the preceding 12 months (Feldman, 1966). Among those who had seen a doctor within the specified period, almost nine-tenths (89 percent) said they were "entirely satisfied." One-tenth (11 percent) were "not entirely satisfied," although this proportion jumped to one-fifth (21 percent) for those with below-average health, the group within which one might expect the elderly to be over-represented.

Over 15 years later, in 1971, NORC carried out another sample survey of how the civilian noninstitutionalized U.S. population viewed their medical care in the midst of what some believed was a "crisis in medical care" (Andersen, Kravitz, & Anderson, 1971). Assessing the medical care the head of the family and those close to him or her had received over the past few years, one-tenth (10 percent) of the family heads expressed dissatisfaction with the quality of medical care received. Among those aged 65 and over, the proportion dissatisfied was less than in the general population. The dissatisfied ranged from 2 percent of the elderly who were nonwhite and not poor, to 10 percent of those elderly who were both nonwhite and poor. There was very little difference in the proportion dissatisfied between the elderly white poor (5 percent) and the elderly white nonpoor (4 percent). Over one-third of the general public and of the elderly were dissatisfied with the cost of care, with waiting time in doctors' office or clinics, and with availability of medical care at night and on weekends (Andersen, Kravitz, & Anderson, 1971). But less than one-tenth (8 percent) of the public registered dissatisfaction with the courtesy and consideration shown by doctors and nurses; among the elderly, the proportions dissatisfied with these features of care were even less, reaching a maximum of 6 percent for poor nonwhite persons.

The most recent NORC survey, directed by the Center for Health Administration Studies of the University of Chicago and sponsored by The Robert Wood Johnson Foundation (1978), was conducted in 1975–1976. The proportion of the noninstitutionalized population who were dissatisfied with the quality of care they had received in a 12-month period was still relatively small (13 percent), though slightly higher than in 1971. Compared with 1971, about the same percentage was dissatisfied with cost of care (37 percent in 1975–1976 vs. 38 percent in 1971) and with the courtesy and consideration shown by doctors and nurses (by doctors: 8 percent dissatisfied in 1975–1976 and 8 percent in 1971; by nurses: 7 percent dissatisfied in 1975–1976, 8 percent in 1971). Dissatisfaction with the waiting time required to see the doctor had declined, from 37 percent in 1971 to 28 percent in 1975–1976. Specific data for the elderly from this survey have not yet been published. Unpublished data (Fleming, n.d.) indicate, however, that other things being equal, expressed dissatisfaction with most dimensions of health care decreases with age: in general, among the noninstitutionalized public, the elderly were more likely to be satisfied than younger age-groups.

Due to the general wording of some of the questions, the extent of satisfaction and dissatisfaction with medical care reflected in these national surveys spanning some twenty years refers to medical care in both outpatient settings (offices and clinics) and in hospitals, except where one or the other setting is specifically indicated (e.g., "office waiting time"). Nevertheless, since in any given year many more persons make visits to the doctor's office or clinic than are hospitalized, it is reasonable to assume that these expressions of opinion apply as much or more to outpatient care than to hospital care. To the extent that this assumption is valid, it would appear that the large majority of the noninstitutionalized public and of the elderly among them have been and are presently generally satisfied with the quality of their office or clinic medical care as they perceive it. However, sizable minorities are dissatisfied with the cost of care and with waiting time required to see the doctor.

Lest these small percentages of dissatisfied people lead to complacency, it is well to remember that in a national survey of the American noninstitutionalized public, even small percentages stand for large numbers of individuals. For example, although "only" 13 percent were dissatisfied with the quality of medical care they received in 1975–1976, this percentage in fact represents over 20 million dissatisified people.

Hospital Care. In a national survey of adults aged 18 and over conducted in 1978 by Harris and associates and sponsored by Hospital Affiliates International, public satisfaction with the quality of care in hospitals was explicitly explored (see also Freidson & Feldman, 1958). In response to a question to be answered in terms of "your own experience and that of your family," nearly one-fifth (18 percent) of the respondents said they were dissatisfied with "the quality of health care to patients staying in hospitals." Among the 16 percent in the sample who had actually been hospitalized within the past year, however, 13 percent were dissatisfied with the quality of care provided by the hospital.

Nevertheless, when asked to rate various features of hospitals as "excellent," "pretty good," "only fair," or "poor," on the basis of their own experience and that of friends and relatives who had been in the hospital, higher proportions of the total sample had specific complaints. About one-sixth (17 percent) rated the care provided by doctors in hospitals as only fair or poor, and one-fifth (20 percent) gave the same low ratings to care provided by nurses in hospitals. Fair or poor ratings were also assigned by one-third (34 percent) of the respondents to the "respect and concern for patients as individuals" shown in hospitals. And a majority (74 percent) gave fair or poor ratings to hospitals on the issue of "charging reasonable fees" (Harris and Associates, 1978).

Although the sample used to generate these findings is described as a "national cross-section of 1503 adults aged 18 and over," of whom 41 percent were aged 50 and over (weighted percentage, 35 percent), the study report unfortunately presents no breakdowns of opinion by age. Thus, we know that a large majority of the U.S. noninstitutionalized population was satisfied with the quality of hospital care in 1978. And we know that many also had specific complaints about certain features of hospitals, most notably costs. But we do not know the extent to which these generalizations apply specifically to the elderly, the age group most likely to be hospitalized.

Nursing Home Care. We badly need information about nursing home residents' satisfaction with their doctors, their medical and nursing care, and with the nursing home itself. One of the few attempts to study residents' reactions to institutional surroundings was the national survey of institutionalized persons (U.S. Bureau of the Census, 1978). Examples of the findings include: 92 percent "like" staff, 91 percent "like" their lodging, 83 percent "like" their meals. Physicians, nurses, and medical care were not asked about explicitly. This manner of inquiry is less than completely satisfactory, since old people, and particularly those in institutions, tend to answer in the most socially acceptable fashion. We clearly need more and better exploration of such evaluations by the consumers of service, including information about their satisfaction with *medical* care received.

Technical Quality of Care

We turn now to a very brief overview of what we know about the technical quality of medical care in the three settings.

It is necesary to say first that wide variations in quality of care as measured by process or outcome variables have been known to occur in structurally similar settings. And structurally dissimilar qualifications and settings do not always show the differences in process or outcome quality that might be expected. Consequently, it has appeared to many investigators that the most appropriate use of the structural approach in assessing the technical quality of care is to recognize that structural factors such as physician qualifications, staffing patterns, and physical facilities may promote or hinder good medical care, in the sense of being important preconditions (Donabedian, 1966; Goss, 1970; Palmer & Reilly, 1979). Thus, they bear investigation in their own right, as licensing and accrediting agencies have recognized for a long time. But they do not substitute for studies of how care is in fact delivered (process) or its effect on patients' health (clinical outcome).

However, all of the studies of the clinical process or outcome of medical care carried out thus far have been exceedingly limited as to time, place, and focus; in many studies little or no attention has been given to proper sampling so as to permit generalization to a larger population (Brook & Williams, 1975; Donabedian, 1978). As a result, what we know about the quality of care in hospitals and in doctors' offices or clinics in the United States is based on relatively small-scale studies conducted sporadically over the past few decades (Palmer & Reilly, 1979). Further, a great deal more attention has been given to evaluating the quality of medical care in hospitals than in doctors' offices or clinics. Even less attention has been given to nursing homes in this respect.

Nevertheless, within the limits of available knowledge it is safe to say that the quality of medical care in outpatient settings and hospitals appears to be variable, and that the variability does not seem to be random. Rather, there is what Donabedian (1977) has called an "epidemiology" of poor (or good) medical care; poor technical quality is more often seen in certain subtypes of each setting, and in certain types of physicians than in others.

Medical Care in Hospitals. In the case of hospitals, there is scattered evidence to suggest that patients are likely to receive better medical care in teaching hospitals, and especially in medical-school-affiliated teaching hospitals; in nonprofit hospitals; in hospitals where high volumes of patients are treated for the illness or condition in question; and in hospitals with an organized, specialized medical staff, at least some of whom are salaried (Palmer & Reilly, 1979).

But even in the "best" hospitals, some poor care may be found; and in hospitals without the characteristics just listed, some very good care has been documented. And, while board-certified specialists have been shown to give better care in their specialty than generalists, the specialists who practice in medical-school-affiliated teaching hospitals are more likely to deliver good care than their specialist counterparts who function in other types of hospitals (Palmer & Reilly, 1979).

Accreditation by the Joint Commission on Accreditation of Hospitals does not appear to be closely related to the quality of hospital care as indicated by process or outcome studies (Goss, 1970). Possibly this represents a "ceiling effect," in that the large majority of hospitals in the United States are now accredited.

Medical Care in Offices/Clinics. We unfortunately still know very little about the quality of office and clinic care, especially when care in physicians' private offices or small group practices is considered. Comparative studies of private office practice are still in their infancy, in part because the records private practitioners keep—when they keep them—do not lend themselves easily to routine coding and analysis, and also because some physicians are reluctant to share the information in their records or to be observed. Nevertheless, one observational study of a sample of general practitioners in North Carolina carried out over 20 years ago showed about two-fifths of the doctors performing at an unsatisfactory level. Better performance correlated with laboratory access, office appointment systems, younger age, and training beyond internship in internal medicine, but not with income, school of graduation, or medical school class rank (Peterson et al., 1956). Other studies suggest that the technical quality of care may be higher in group practice than in solo general practice, and that neighborhood health centers may provide as good or better care than teaching hospital outpatient clinics (Palmer & Reilly, 1979).

In neither hospital nor outpatient quality-of-care studies has much attention been paid to the technical quality of care given to the elderly, as this might differ from that given other categories of patients in each setting. To the extent that the elderly represent an economically and otherwise disadvantaged group, however, the conclusion of a careful survey of research reported by Brook and Williams (1975:132) is worth quoting: "The quality of health care for the disadvantaged is not strikingly poorer than the care for the nondisadvantaged, but, in view of demonstrable shortcomings in the quality of health care in general, this is not viewed as a positive statement." Further, one study of quality care in hospitals in Hawaii found "no overall consistent evidence that hospitalized elderly patients were treated by their physicians with a different level of personal medical care than were younger adult patients" (Lyons & Payne, 1974:337). Coe and Brehm (1972), however, found certain deficiencies in the preventive care provided to older adults in the offices of general practitioners and internists.

Medical Care in Nursing Homes. Assessments of quality of care in nursing homes have been based more often on structural characteristics of homes, such as staffing patterns and cleanliness of patients' rooms, than on process-of-care or outcome-of-care variables (Abdellah, 1977; Kart & Manard, 1976). And studies that have focused on these latter types of variables have been more concerned with the process of nursing care and the outcomes of nursing care than with processes and outcomes of medical care as such. An admirable recent study (Linn, Gurel, & Linn, 1977) of patient outcomes over a six-month period as a measure of quality of nursing home care, for example, examines three outcome variables: mortality, change in functional status (improved, unchanged, deteriorated), and change in patient location (discharged, still in nursing home, readmitted to hospital). In attempting to characterize homes with better outcomes, the investigators examined numerous features of the 40 homes involved in the study. A major conclusion was that "homes with more RN hours per patient were associated with patients being alive, improved, and discharged from the home." They arrived at this conclusion, however, without taking into account possible variations in physician care of the patients that might help account for the different outcomes.

It may well be that the quality of medical care provided by physicians is much less relevant to how patients fare in nursing homes than in short-term hospitals. Certainly, the two settings have different concentrations of patients with diagnoses in which improvement—or even survival—can be expected. But we presently know very little about physician care in nursing homes on a systematic basis. One suggestive study by Gottesman and Boureston (1974) observed ongoing behavior in a sample of 44 nursing homes on 27,000 patient occasions. In only 2 percent of these occasions did the investigators observe any behavior that could be categorized as medical or nursing treatment; they did not evaluate the quality of treatment provided. It would now be eminently worthwhile to go beyond existing research to assess the technical quality of both nursing and medical care separately. In such research a somewhat different perspective on quality than has been developed for evaluating hospital or office or clinic care may be called for, of course. But the task does not seem impossible (see, e.g., Donabedian, 1978; Plant, 1977), and, if undertaken, could yield large dividends.

Summary

In summary, national sample surveys of the U.S. noninstitutionalized population have told us quite a bit about how satisfied people in general and the elderly in particular are with the care they receive in doctors' offices and clinics. But relatively little is known about the technical quality of the medical care actually delivered in these outpatient settings. More—though far from enough—information exists concerning the technical quality of medical care delivered in short-term hospitals. Also, public satisfaction with care in hospitals has been explored in a recent national sample survey of the noninstitutionalized U.S. population. Patients' satisfaction with care in nursing homes has never been studied on a national basis, however, and the technical quality of medical care that nursing home patients receive remains essentially unassessed and unknown. Unfortunately, patients in nursing homes are also the group with the least control over and in their relationships with doctors. Others must, therefore, speak for them if they are to benefit from current concerns with the aged, with "consumerism," and with professional "accountability." Well-designed research on the quality of medical care received by nursing-home patients, as indicated by technical as well as psychological outcomes, is clearly needed as a basis for informed social policy in the years to come. The time to begin the research is now.

14
Strategies of Power and Dependence in Doctor-Patient Exchanges

SAMUEL W. BLOOM, Ph.D., AND
EDWARD J. SPEEDLING, Ph.D.

Introduction

The ability to influence others is the essence of all power, and its tools are control and authority. There are, however, distinctly different levels of social behavior for the application of power concepts: the microlevel of interpersonal relations and the macrolevel, shaped by interaction between classes, interest groups, and institutions (Coser & Larsen, 1976).

In the sociology of medicine, the role of the professional as an agent of social control and related issues of authority have been central for more than half a century, beginning with the analysis of the doctor-patient relationship in the early work of Henderson (1935) and Parsons (1951). Their approach focused on the interpersonal level and was, therefore, essentially social-psychological, oriented toward explaining social action and the social roles of the individual actors. Analytically, they were concerned about how the institutions of medicine and the structure of society shaped the patterns of interaction between professionals and their clients; but the center of inquiry was at the microlevel of social interaction. What happens, they asked, between the doctor and patient? The patterns of such relations, they believed, represented the structure of the society; and the substance reflected the culture, learned through socialization.

More recently—about 10 years ago, to be more precise—the literature of medical sociology took a distinct turn in its approach to issues of power. Actually, Eliot Freidson's first book on medicine, published in 1961, presaged the direction, but it was not until his later books on professional dominance and autonomy (1970b, 1970c) followed by a series of studies on the political economy of health (Ehrenreich & Ehrenreich, 1970; Stevens, 1971;

Waitzkin & Waterman, 1974; Navarro, 1976; Illich, 1975; Krause, 1977) that a full-blown political sociology of health and medical care was established in the United States. These books were about classes and interest groups, studying what Coser calls their "relational aspects" (Coser, 1976:334).[1]

In selecting an approach that has particular relevance to the elderly patient, we have decided to limit our discussion to what we know best, focusing at the level of individual social interaction. This should in no way suggest that we think that the relational approach of political sociology is less valuable. It does assert that we believe social interaction theory continues to have something important to say about this subject.

Specific for the elderly patient, the theoretical literature appears currently to be changing from emphasis on variables of types of illness and disability toward a new awareness of the experience of the aged as a constituent group, especially within the institutional frameworks that are provided for them. We argue that the sources of their own losses, their stigmatized status, and their forced dependency—as others in this book have described at length—must be calibrated against the ambiguity of the roles to which they are assigned. In explanation, we will draw on theories of adult socialization. So far, these theories have not elaborated very fully older adulthood as a stage of human growth and development, and this vagueness reflects the normative values of the culture. We attempt to extrapolate from general socialization theory the categories and markers of behavior that must be clarified to understand the experience of the elderly, and perhaps to prevent the alienation and despair that too often is their fate.

Power in Interpersonal Relations: Structures and Strategy

Between professionals and clients in modern western society, the weight of power is one-sided. Doctors, for example, possess monopolistic control over such vital aspects of health care as drugs and hospital access. Theirs is also the authority both of licensure based on extensive professional education and examination and of the prestige and trust that the public assigns to the physicians' presumed expertise. Dependence is reciprocal to power; it is, in its dictionary definition, "the quality or state of being influenced by or subject to another" (*Webster's New Collegiate Dictionary*, 1974:304). The patient appears to be inherently dependent within the situation of doctor-patient exchanges.

Given this basic structure of clearly assigned dominance and subordinateness, wherein does the question of "strategies" arise? Closer scrutiny reveals that the order of power is not as stable as it first appears. Influence varies according to types of illness, age, and social class of the patient, and the organization of health-care delivery. Doctors act to protect their power, often in the name of what they consider the requisites of fulfilling their responsibilities, and patients act to assert what increasingly is socially defined as their "right" to health care.

Discussion of this issue can be found in the very earliest literature of medical sociology. Henderson, in 1935, described the imbalance of the social roles in the doctor-patient relationship. The patient, he said, cannot be expected to be rational or fully in control of self when confronted with the unknowns of the disturbing symptoms of illness. The doctor must calculate the fears and anxieties of the patient, and communicate selectively. Words, Henderson wrote, can wound as deeply as a scalpel, just as they can heal if properly used. The flow of this vital communication, however, was, in Henderson's model, and somewhat contradictory to his basic theory, essentially one-way, from the doctor to the patient. The doctor was in control.

Parsons (1951) elaborated Henderson's social role analysis in his conception of the "asymmetry" of the doctor-patient relationship. The doctor, Parsons emphasized, achieves a status based on "technical specificity," or expert skill and knowledge. The privileges of his professional role are granted because of that expertise. For Parsons, the patient's special privileges in what he called the "sick role" were temporary, and also they represented a risk for the society. Cultural norms prescribe that the patient must "seek expert help" in order to get well and return to his or her appropriate "functioning" normal role. The patient learns about the obligations and privileges of the sick role through the society's structured processes of socialization (especially as institutionalized in the family), and the doctor, within Parsons' model, is the agent of social control for the society to protect both from the threat of illness and the risks of the sick role.

The Henderson-Parsons model is very close to the systems perspective developed by George Engel at the beginning of this book. The papers of Marshall, Maddox, and Coe, on the other hand, develop both the amplifications and some of the criticisms of social system theories that have appeared in the literature. We will avoid repetition by concentrating briefly only on those aspects of previous work that relate to problems of the elderly patient, mainly as the foundation for adding two perspectives that are often less evident: human growth and development as it applies to adult socialization, and sociohistorical cohort analysis.

Behavioral Implications of Organic Symptoms

One of the striking omissions in Parsons is a discussion of how variation in type of illness can directly influence the social behavior of both doctor and patient. He did note that illness is "partly biologically defined" and that the "state of the organism as a biological system" is related to the social systems of medical practice. However, his illustrations on this point tended to concentrate on two types of cases: on sexuality as a threat to the obligation of the doctor to be affectively neutral and on emotional (psychiatric) illness as a special case, different in its implications from physical illness (see Bloom & Wilson, 1979).

Szasz and Hollender (1956) constructed a threefold model of the doctor-patient relationship that corrected for Parsons' omission. Table 14–1 summarizes this model.

The contribution of this model is disarmingly simple. How one can and should behave, as either patient or dictor, varies according to whether the symptoms of illness are acute and disabling, acute and mysterious or distressing even though only mildly disabling, or chronic especially when more or less symptom-free. For the extreme acute organic symptoms, the physi-

TABLE 14–1
Szasz-Hollender Models of the Doctor-Patient Relationship

Model	Physician's Role	Patient's Role	Clinical Application of Model	Prototype of Model
Activity-passivity	Does something to patient	Recipient (unable to respond or inert)	Anesthesia, acute trauma, coma, delirium, etc.	Parent-infant
Guidance-cooperation	Tells patient what to do	Cooperator (obeys)	Acute infectious processes, etc.	Parent-child (adolescent)
Mutual participation	Helps patient to help himself	Participant in "partnership" (uses expert help)	Most chronic illnesses, psychoanalysis, etc.	Adult-adult

Source: Szasz & Hollender, 1956.

cian obviously must take charge, and the patient cannot question. For the less extreme condition, an authoritarian posture by the physician can create resistance where cooperation is needed. In the chronic condition, such as diabetes mellitus, the patient must become an equal participant in treatment, requiring the physician to be a treatment-partner rather than the active giver to a passive recipient.

For the discussion here, there are several important observations to be made from the Szasz-Hollender model. Clearly, "strategies" of power and dependence are highlighted and explained. For the elderly, chronic illness is demonstrably more likely to become a major problem of existence. How does the medical profession respond? Is it the main "strategy" of physicians to educate and facilitate mutual cooperation with their elderly patients? In other words, do physicians encourage *in*dependence in their chronically ill elderly patients (or is it more characteristic to feed their feelings of *dependence*)? What, in turn, are the powers of the elderly in such situations? Can they assert a will to independence, toward maximum control over their own lives? Or are they either directly or indirectly forced into behaviors of passivity, able to express their frustrations only through passive forms of aggression? The Szasz-Hollender model is useful, we believe, in clarifying a range of problems that emerge from the behavioral implications of organic symptoms.

The weakness of the model derives from its reliance, like system analysis, on a conception of inherent asymmetry, with the physician dominant. It leans heavily on the parent-child analogy with explicit role differences that, in effect, always retain control in the hands of the professional, and cast the patient in a childlike status. For the elderly, this can only feed the "second-childhood" stereotype. It is, finally, limited to social psychological analysis, and therefore, though valid at that level, it does not account for variables in the structure of the treatment situation (e.g., private fee-for-service vs. prepaid group practice or other more bureaucratized delivery of care) or for external variables such as socioeconomic status, gender, or age-related status.

Freidson, for example, has argued that the Parsonian analysis of role is incomplete because it does not account for the constituent groups—the lay referral network of the patient and the professional network of the physician. Instead of the doctor and patient acting according to cultural expectations, Freidson sees each role determined by the interests deriving from different and necessarily conflicting social perspectives. The particular professional-client encounter *negotiates* these interests, he says, rather than simply fulfilling the functional requisites of the social system.

McKinlay adds the conception of a series of "counterpositions" that must be negotiated simultaneously. Thus, as shown in Figure 14–1, a patient, in the sick role, must engage spouse and work colleagues as well as the health professional. Each of these critical role partners is inevitably involved in the consequences of illness, and each acts from a different perspective. Indeed, and this is particularly imminent in the situation of the elderly patient, the sick role is often and sometimes necessarily negotiated in a *triadic* relationship, rather than the dyad of doctor and patient. For example, a son or daughter may assume the responsibility for an elderly patient, communicating with the doctor for the patient and determining what treatment decisions will be made in the immediate and the long term. No matter how sincerely the patient's offspring may try to represent the interests of the parent ("acting in the best interests of the parent" is the popular phrase), it

FIGURE 14–1
Counterpositions to Be Negotiated Simultaneously by the Patient

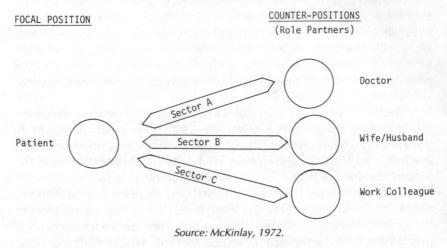

FOCAL POSITION   COUNTER-POSITIONS
                                                         (Role Partners)

Patient   Sector A   Doctor

                   Sector B   Wife/Husband

                   Sector C   Work Colleague

Source: McKinlay, 1972.

requires no stretch of the imagination to recognize that the perspectives of child and parent in such a situation may conflict. Irving Rosow's presentation in this book concerning the triads that typify the treatment sitaution of elderly patients, and the coalitions that result, has made this dramatically clear.

The Power Factors

At this point, three distinct types of behavior have been introduced into the discussion, each of which varies on a continuum:

1. acute–chronic (symptoms)
2. dependent–independent (sick role response)
3. powerless–powerful (situational status)

In combination, the first two form the models of doctor-patient relationships described by Szasz-Hollender. The third is added by Freidson, and is used to reject the basic assumption of asymmetry and social system, replacing them with the concept of a *negotiated* order of unstable *superordinacy-subordinacy*. With this revision, issues of dominance and monopoly are introduced. The frame of reference of social system theory is replaced with the model of the marketplace.

To illustrate, the elderly patient, according to the functional social system model, typically enters the health-care system because of chronic illness. Acute episodes will occur, but chronic degenerative problems are most prevalent. Does the health system deal with these problems on an individual basis according to the psychological dynamics described by Szasz-Hollender, or are labels applied and cost-benefit ratios used to decide vital questions of treatment? What are the cultural values that apply, and how do they affect the elderly patient? Is it possible that one of the reasons for the urgency, the stridency of our statements about the aged, is the fact that the society as a whole has stigmatized the aged with the prognostic labels "troublesome," "unproductive," and "incurable"? Have we not medicalized the normal problems of aging in order to create a new marketplace of medical care commodities, utilizing Medicare, pension plans, and insurance to commercialize values that supersede the humanitarian ethics traditionally associated with medical care? Is it possible that these tendencies are at the source of the heightened political concern about cost, scarcity, productivity, and cost benefits in our national policy about health care at this time? If the answer to these questions is affirmative, and we assert here that it is, the next question is how have we arrived at these attitudes?

We will not attempt to deal fully with so complex a problem in the limited space still available, but let us set what we believe will be a healthful direction for inquiry.

Socialization Theory:[2]
Some Applications to Problems of Aging

Socialization is a broad term for the whole process by which an individual, born with behavioral potentialities of enormously wide range, is led to develop actual behavior that is confined within a much narrower range—the scope of what is customary and acceptable for him according to the standards of his group (Child, 1954:655). In early usage, it was viewed almost entirely as a childhood process. The work of anthropologists brought into focus the patterned variations of behavior in whole societies and, together with psychologists, found the explanations in child-rearing practices. Conceptually, the key assumption is that the individual internalizes from current experience standards of future conduct. Moreover, these internalizations in personality are believed to be stable and long lasting, the framework for more or less automatic reactions to the choices of behavior that are part of everyday experience.

For a long time, socialization was distinguished from other forms of learning by time of life, a process mainly of the early years of infancy and childhood. Later learning was "education." One's attitudes and values, in other words, were essentially established in the family, acting as the socializing institution of the society, and knowledge and skills were acquired in educational institutions, as a kind of superstructure of the person. It is generally accepted today that such earlier assumptions were too rigidly tied to the childhood hypothesis. Character, the structure of personality that phrases the individual's assimilation of social tradition, is no longer assumed to be set in the concrete of early life. Character can and does, the adult socialization hypothesis argues, develop and change throughout life.

Acknowledging, however, that socialization is a lifelong process does not mean that it is the same throughout. There are developmental requirements associated with the phases of life, and the patterns of socialization are their reflections. If we look at the *content* of socialization, for example, in the infant the concentration of developmental thrust is organic, and socialization deals mainly with feeding, nurturing, and in general, controlling the body. The consequences of varying culture are vividly illustrated in anthropological examples that show how child-rearing practices can influence the membership of a whole human society toward (or against) generosity, obsessiveness, and sexuality. As the infant grows into childhood, there is a shift toward psychological development, culminating in the identity formation of adolescence. Before adulthood, the psychological integration of a whole self is assumed to have taken place. In adulthood, therefore, the emphasis of adaptation shifts from the intrapsychic toward the interpersonal and sociocultural.

Content is only one basis for distinguishing the phases of socialization, however. Patterned changes occur in various characteristics, as shown in Table 14–2, and on these bases, age-graded profiles can be described. The profile of childhood, in addition to focusing on the control and integration of biological growth, is involved in rapid learning of the completely new materials of experience. Civilization has arranged for this to occur mainly in protected environments, so that the first steps in the awakening of a self tend to be idealized, and, removed from reality pressures; the child is more idealistic at this stage than he will be in adulthood. "Don't be a child!" or "Don't be naïve!" we say to the adult idealist.

Similarly, if we analyze the social role, the child is characteristically subordinate in status: the dependent of adult parents or the neophyte student of adult teachers. There is a strong emotional charge in these relationships, intensified by the no-escape situational structure of required memberships in family and school and the restricted access to the social world that age places on the child.

How does this approach apply to aging? And, to strategies of power and dependence in doctor-patient exchanges involving the elderly patient?

First, we propose that the elderly represent a stage in human growth and development that can be demarcated in similar terms to the other stages shown in Table 14–2. We call this stage *advanced adulthood*, a term that avoids stigma but retains the integrity of separateness much the same

TABLE 14–2

Socialization Differences in Childhood, Adolescence, and Adulthood*

Basis of Distinctions	Childhood	Adolescence	Adulthood
Content	Regulation of biological drives	Develop overarching values, self-image	Overt norms and behaviors (work role), more superficial personality traits
Involvement	Learning new material; more idealistic because situation removed from daily pressures		More realistic; synthesis of previously learned; reconciles contradictory norms
Social role	Dependent, student	Dependent, student, peer	Student or apprentice; full role incumbent (worker, spouse, parent)
Context	Family, school	Family, school, peer group	Occupational group or its training institution, own family
Socializer/ socializee relationship		Emotionally charged	More formalized
Structure of situation	Required membership in family and school; restricted to small peer group		In position to withdraw, to initiate changes of career, divorce, etc.; responsible within role set
Learner-socializee response	Malleable to group norms	Conflicted, ambivalent but malleable	Resistant to psychological change. Self-interest can lead to conformity or independent challenge of group norms

*This table was created by adapting the types and patterns of socialization described in Mortimer & Simmons, 1978.

as Levinson's "early adult transition" (Levinson, 1978:21–138). Our "advanced adulthood" may be marked for entry by age 65, the normal qualifying year for Social Security, and continue to the end of life.[3] Like Levinson's "novicehood," it should be divided into subcategories; but, for the moment, we discuss it as a single general stage.

The transition into advanced adulthood obviously involves dramatic changes in role expectation. This statement applies equally to the other major life cycle transitions, but this, the final stage of life, contains very specific differentiating qualities. It is, generally, different from what Lowenthal and her associates call the "incremental" transitions —becoming a person, leaving home, and starting a family (Lowenthal et al., 1975). It is "decremental," typified by problems of reduction and loss—continuing the earlier emptying of the family nest, reducing work commitments, and dealing with the death of friends, spouse, self.

More precisely, using the categories we developed earlier, advanced adulthood can be summarized as in Table 14–3. Studying this portrait, one is reminded of Benedict's observation that some sequential age roles are sharply discontinuous (Benedict, 1938). For example, the child is socialized to be nonresponsible, submissive, and asexual, while the adult is expected to be responsible, dominant, and sexually active. To accomplish this transition, socialization after childhood is necessary, as Mortimer and Simmons (1978) discuss at length. The same authors describe a similarly dramatic discontinuity in the reverse direction at the end of the life cycle:

> Throughout adult life, autonomy and productivity have been emphasized, particularly for men. Work and achievement have been paramount to the self-image of the adult male and to his role within the family. Yet, when retirement comes, this central work role is suddenly lost (Cavan, 1971; Bengston & Haber, 1975), and the husband becomes a part-time housekeeper along with his wife (Lipman, 1961). With advancing age, health and financial problems cause greater dependency, sometimes to the point of institutionalization (Tissue, 1970). *There is comparatively little preparation for such fundamental life change.* [our emphasis, from Mortimer & Simmons, 1978:425]

TABLE 14–3
Socialization: Advanced Adulthood

Content	Management of the biological change of aging, and the loss of central work role; adaptation of self-image from centrality of work-achievement to "retirement"; maintenance of integrity of self in the face of nearness of "not being."
Involvement	Realistic; the summary and refinement of all that was previously learned with a framework of altered capabilities; the renunciation of unachieved or no-longer-feasible life goals and the achievement of wisdom (Erikson, 1959).
Social role	The Elder; in American society, this typically involves role reversal, withdrawal to less central and less important status; retiree; part-time worker and/or housekeeper; dependent; potential client for special institutions for the old; widow/widower.
Context	Family; special communities for aged; special institutions for aged.
Socializer/ socializee relationship	Emotionally charged; reversal of relationship with children, employer, professionals.
Structure of situations	Ambiguous in family, work environments, and special institutions.
Learner-socializee response	Wisdom can lead to generativity, the helping of younger former subordinates; alienation can lead to ritual compliance with social norms, bitter passive resistance, or withdrawal into invalidism.

It is important to add that *the styles of coping with life changes are dramatically different for men and women* (Lowenthal, 1975).

Two critical summary conclusions should be inserted at this point in the discussion:

1. The sequences of age roles from adulthood to advanced adulthood (old age) are sharply discontinuous.
2. This requires socialization *after* entrance into the latter stage.

If we are effectively to accomplish such socialization, there is a set of criteria that are proposed for the facilitation of the process (Mortimer & Simmons, 1978:425)):

- There should be "normative clarity," a focus on clear, visible roles.
- Transitions from prior roles should be institutionalized and accompanied by clear "rites of passage."
- Rituals making the role transitions are important.
- The major role should be highly visible to nonincumbents.
- The new role should be compatible with other concurrent roles.

Not only does our society provide very little institutionalized socialization for the final stage of aging, but the ambiguity of its role definitions undercuts the effectiveness of those patterns that exist.

Sociohistorical Cohorts

There are several prevailing frameworks within which the adaptive processes of adulthood have been studied. Perhaps best known is the psychodynamic concept of "the ever-recurring life plot," which is entrenched in Freud (Fromm, 1966, cited in Lowenthal et al., 1975). There is also a traditional view of sociology in which social structure is viewed as the major source of differences between life-stage or age cohorts. Finally, there are psychocultural conceptions, identified mainly with Erikson (1959, 1963, 1968), and sometimes called theories of self-actualization (Lowenthal,1975).

There is the danger in all these perspectives of a too-static conception of stages of the life course, a cross-sectional view that does not account for important changes that are part of social history. Matilda Riley and her collaborators (Riley et al., 1969; Riley, Johnson, & Foner, 1972) have in recent years developed and documented the arguments of cohort analysis.

Cohort analysis, on the one hand, has described specific structural factors that change over time, such as life expectation, and interpreted their effects on life experience. The most basic demographic fact is the growth of the proportion of the population aged 65 and above. Related to this general statistic are a variety of specific events. For example, median age of widow-hood increased almost 8 years, from 53.3 to 60.9, during the 50 years be-tween 1890 and 1940. This rate of increase has been sustained since, passing 65 in 1980. Each decade has produced a cohort that has a different expe-rience of the age of death of spouse (Neugarten, Moore, & Lowe, 1968).At the same time, labor force participation has decreased among older adults. In 1947, the population of men aged 65 and over in the labor force was 48 per-cent; in 1957, 38 percent; in 1966, only 27 percent (U..S. Department of La-bor, 1967:202). Thus, we know that each successive cohort of older male Americans has been larger in total size but smaller in proportion remaining in the labor force. Stated more simply, the most fundamental aspects of life —love as expressed in marriage and work—have changed for each succes-sive age cohort of this century.

In addition to such structural changes, however, critical historical ex-perience varies. If we change the four major life stages, by 20-year birth co-horts, listing the major events of each historical period, the result can be diagrammed. Table 14–4 illustrates how different the experience of a given stage of life is for successive age cohorts. The child of 1900 grew up in a radi-cally different social environment from the child of 1920 or 1930 or 1970. To grow up in a world dominated by small towns but with all the optimistic thrust of the technological revolution at the turn of the century contrasts with the childhood dominated by fear of atomic holocaust, of uncertainties about the human capacity to control a runaway technology. Therefore, the group that is in the advanced adult stage today cannot be used as a model for the group that will enter this stage in one or two decades. One of the conse-quences of this fact is keenly evident in the requirements of socialization for advanced adulthood.

Summary and Conclusions

When theories of adult socialization process and sociohistorical analysis are integrated in reformulating the problem of aging in America, one sees the persistence of cultural attitudes that were appropriate 50 years ago unyield-ing to radically altered social conditions of the present. Individualism, self-reliance, postponement of gratification for future rewards—these are the cultural values that were the foundations on which the present cohort of el-derly Americans prepared for their old age, and these same values continue to grip the imagination of the society. Such values place the burden of adap-tation on the internal psychological resources of the aged individual, but in a changed environment that lacks both functional roles and appropriate insti-tutions for the elderly.

TABLE 14—4
Major Historical Events of the Twentieth Century in the United States
According to the Stages of the Life Cycle of 20-Year Cohorts

Birth Cohort	Life Stages			
	Childhood	Adolescence	Adulthood	Old Age
Pre–1900	Scientific revolution; frontier conquest	Depression; Spanish-American War; American isolationism	World War I; boom/bust economy	World War II; Cold War and expanding postwar economy
1900-1919	Peaceful Teddy Roosevelt decade	World War I	Boom 1920s; Depression; World War II; Cold War	Civil rights movement; Viet Nam War; stagflation
1920–1939	Boom economy optimism	Depression; New Deal	World War II; McCarthy era; economic expansion	Uncertainties of economy and environment; expanded numbers of elderly
1940–1959	World War II; atomic bomb	Korean War; McCarthy era; hydrogen bomb	Civil rights movement; Viet Nam War; stagflation; population explosion; fear for the environment; energy crisis	
1960–1979	Space age; civil rights movement; Viet Nam War	Sexual revolution; stagflation; Watergate		

In the individual encounter between the physician and the elderly patient, the result is a situation of ambiguous role expectations, a poor fit with the structural elements of modern society. Each criticizes the other in terms of old voluntaristic values from the age of individualism, but each is constrained by conditions that promote collective action: the runaway costs that make obsolete the responsibility of individuals for the costs of their own medical care, the expanded technology that forces physicians out of entrepreneurial and into bureaucratized organizations of health-care delivery. It is against this background that issues of power and dependence in the doctor-patient encounter must be studied.

In this presentation, we have taken the opportunity to develop freely a broad array of themes so that our conclusions can only be suggested. The power of the physician, certainly, does not appear to be as firmly legitimized as it was 50 years ago. The basis of that power, explained in the social psychology of interpersonal relations, was valid for the conditions that prevailed when Henderson and Parsons first presented that type of conceptual framework. However, those conditions have changed, forcing the negotiation of power between doctor and patient to shift from individual to collective premises. The contemporary languages of power involve the constraints of law, of professional standards, of consumers' rights, instead of their previous focus on transactions at the level of interaction process. Both levels are still operative, but the current realities press for attention more to the sociopolitical than to the social psychological.

Notes

1. Although Coser (1976) was discussing stratification, his point is valid for the distinction we are making here. He distinguished between *distributive* and *relational* aspects of social class. The former focuses "predominantly on the impact on individual careers of differences in parental resources, access to educational institutions and the like, or they center attention upon individual characteristics of people variously placed in the social structure. . . . Yet," Coser adds, "a class system is not only a distributive system, in which individuals are assigned to their respective niches in terms of background and training . . . it is also a system that is shaped by the interaction between various classes and interest groups differentially located within the social structure. It is a system, moreover, in which command and coercion play major parts." Coser uses the following medical illustration: "It is one thing to investigate the ways in which, for example, people manage to attain the status position of medical practitioners in American society; it is quite another to analyze the institutions that help the American Medical Association to monopolize the market for health care by restricting access" (pp. 334–335).
2. This section, in part, is extracted from a longer presentation of the basic conception by one of the authors (Bloom), "The Impact of Medical Education on the Medical Student: A Summary and Evaluation of the State of Knowledge about Socialization for the Profession," Harvard Medical School Symposium on medical education, Sept. 29, 1979, unpublished manuscript.
3. Rose (1968) states, "The age sixty-five has more or less come to be considered as the age of entering old age in American society." He credits the Social Security Act of 1935 and the double exemption of income tax, both setting sixty-five as the age of effectuation, as the events that have made into legal definiton what formerly was only a social category.

PART VI

IMPLICATIONS FOR THE FUTURE

A practicing physician and a gerontologist review the chapters in this book and offer their perspectives on implications for medical practice and research needs. Dr. Ford, a physician with expertise in geriatrics, sees several major issue areas relating to practice, particularly with respect to medical education as undergirding service delivery, and institutional or "quaternary" care. Focusing on stereotyping as a source of shortcomings, Ford makes a strong case for modifications in medical education as a precondition for improvements in the practice of medical care for the elderly, difficult as such modifications may be in light of the constraints built into the educational system. His strong comments in this regard are in harmony with national goals regarding education in geriatrics as seen by institutions like the Academy of Medicine and the National Institute on Aging. Inevitably, he moves into the need for research, posing a whole series of questions about nursing homes, health-care costs, and the impact of political and environmental changes. Also relevant to practice are unanswered questions on how older people define health and on the nature of their health maintenance activities. In short, thinking about practice implications leads to an assessment of current gaps in empirical data and the ways in which the availability of such data would improve the quality of care.

Similarly, although Dr. Lawton, the environmental psychologist with expertise in gerontology, takes as his task an evaluation of present research needs, recognition of the origin in and the interlock of these issues with practice is inescapable. A number of fruitful research leads emerge from Lawton's discussion. Indeed, the fact that he is a psychologist adds a new perspective to the approaches taken elsewhere in the volume. Among the multitude of ideas he offers, several stand out with particular cogency. A basic question with respect to patients concerns their preference for dependence versus independence and its relationship to the level of autonomy sought in interaction with physicians. Ageism in medical practitioners can be studied in terms of the "just world" ideology, which assumes that people get what they deserve, so that decline and loss among the elderly is viewed as an appropriate fate. The actual encounter between aged patients and physicians is another understudied area, which calls for imaginative research methods to uncover factors related to compliance and noncompliance with recommended regimens. The results of all these types of studies would have repercussions for the way medicine is practiced and the way patients, including the elderly, are treated.

This book, then, ends not with definitive answers, but with some of the most important questions. Both physicians and social scientists, however, will find sufficient sustenance for their own interests, specialized and interlocking. As Ford points out, some interdisciplinary misperceptions may be erased and new understanding created concerning what must be a mutual enterprise, achieving quality, satisfactory health care for the elderly.

15
Implications for Practice

AMASA B. FORD, M.D.

Models are clearly important to the issue of the physician-patient relationship. Recognition of this fact reminded me of our middle son, home from college, cleaning out his closet. Out of the depths came a number of partially completed airplane models and several kits that had not even been opened. He decided that these models had been an intense interest of his at one time, but that he had outgrown them, so they went into the rubbish. It made me think that, at the right time, model building can be an effective educational tool. Even though they may be discarded—and we know that some of the earlier models of the doctor-patient relationship have been discarded —models have heuristic and educational value, and they are certainly thought provoking.

One model that may have been discarded can be described, in my view, as the social scientist's view of the physician—autocratic, pompous, and egotistical. I hope that this is one of the stereotypes that can be discarded on the basis of the content of the chapters in this book. Another model may be called the physician's idea of the family and the patient: incompetent, lost, not knowing where to turn. Research data tells us that this, too, is a stereotype and that the family in fact provides much support and strength.

For this final discussion on implications for practice, I would like to touch briefly on three issues relating to practice:

1. medical education, which can be thought of as a form of practice, or certainly an undergirding of practice,
2. primary care, and
3. what may be called quaternary care.

Primary, secondary, and tertiary care are familiar, but tertiary care really does not cover the nursing home and the institution, the places where we find so many old people.

First, in medical education, Engel (Chapter 1) points out that the medical perspective tends to be much too narrow. Maddox (Chapter 6) reminds us that the medical outlook can be too confined, that it tends to be focused in

173

doctors' offices and hospitals and not in other sites where old people live and may be institutionalized. We need to enlarge the curriculum; we must put a lot more into the medical mind and medical perception before we can have a satisfactory doctor. This is a demand that is going to be very hard to meet. The typical medical school's curriculum is inflexible and the curriculum committee not eager to make room for more behavioral science, more sociology, or more opportunities for the medical students to work with the team, despite the fact that these are clearly needed. The solution to this problem perhaps should take the form of a question: How can we get this necessary broadening into the course of medical education? How can we make opportunities for medical students to work with others?

A place to begin may be for scholars and health professionals to show that we can respect each other and work together. A story that Mark Twain used to tell may be apropos. It was about the man who died and was on his way to heaven. As he got closer to the pearly gates, he saw that the gates were a bit ajar. He was waiting outside heaven to go through various bureaucratic procedures, and he said to St. Peter, "Look, I may not even get in here, but could you just push the door open a bit and let me have a look?" St. Peter was very busy, but he agreed, and said he would open it a little. As the man looked inside, he saw an elderly personage with a long white beard pacing up and down with a worried look, wearing a stethoscope around his neck. The man said, "What is going on? I thought in heaven there was no sickness and no suffering, so how can you explain this person I see here?" St. Peter looked over his shoulder and said, "Oh, that's God—sometimes he likes to play at being a doctor!"

Some may indeed have a notion that doctors like to play God. Some physicians also believe that sociologists and "soft" scientists do not have much to contribute. I hope that we can all set aside these misapprehensions and stereotypes. For instance, if there are readers who have doubted that physicians can be dedicated and willing to accept the difficult task of the care of the elderly, I hope they have been impressed by the ideas presented by Williams, Weiss, Breslau, and others in this book. There is much to learn from the issues Williams (Chapter 4) articulates: the spectrum of complaints, multiple conditions, and the other special characteristics of sick old people. The importance of small gains that Weiss (Chapter 8) emphasizes is also extremely important. For many aged, our microscopes must be focused differently; there are special criteria of success in long-term care.

Still, we must alter medical education if we are going to produce enough compassionate and informed physicians. How can we achieve an improvement in health manpower? There are not enough geriatricians. A curious paradox is that the Beeson Committee recommends a specialty of geriatric medicine not be established, and yet recommends that there be a marked increase in teaching and research in geriatric medicine in medical school (Institute of Medicine, 1978). It is not clear where the teachers will come from to do that unless we have a specialty of geriatric medicine. We need better and more accessible model-care situations for teaching. Frankly, there are very few nursing homes that deserve the status of models to medical, nursing, and social work students. Many constraints are built into the system in the quality and availablility of teaching sites. Another educational problem is how to solve the riddle of achieving interdisciplinary education, starting from a certain amount of conflict. There is conflict between the critics of the system and the people struggling with it on the front line. It is not easy to put together multidisciplinary teaching programs with medicine, nursing, and social work students learning side by side. The institutions are not ready, the students are at different levels, territoriality is a problem, and there are financial disincentives that prevent paying for the multidisciplinary team. So we have major needs in medical education and major problems in trying to meet them.

In primary care, Marshall (Chapter 9) refers to negotiating and bargaining as the process of establishing the doctor-patient relationship. What about the concept of the doctor-patient relationship as a contract? Do we really need contracts as a means of proceeding in an interpersonal professional relationship? Do we need contracts in medicine more explicitly than we have them? The recent rise in family medicine is a very important development in geriatric medicine. Continuity of care, one physician, a comprehensive analysis of the patient's needs, and working with a multidisciplinary team all fit perfectly with the needs of elderly people.

Quarternary care is nursing home care. Several vivid pictures have been presented of the continued stress imposed upon the caretakers. Who should carry the responsibility for the care of the institutionalized elderly? Even though we should perhaps move away from the teaching hospital and the intensive institutional teaching situation, we have to admit that this situation exists partly because our high technology has made it possible for more elderly people to survive with more severe disabilities. Prolongation of life becomes a problem. Who is going to carry this responsibility, and how are we going to help the caretakers? We cannot expect family and friends to do it all. Often, a family with a severely disabled older member may reach its limit. Is nursing home care neglected by physicians because it does not pay? Maybe that is one of the major reasons doctors do not go into nursing homes. How can we deal with the demographic facts of more old-old, more senile dementia, more terminal cancer patients with a diminishing supply of potential care givers in the labor market?

Turning now to research, it is exciting to find that there is much evolution toward more appropriate and less rigid models than the ones found 15 years ago. Although Fine (Chapter 5) is the only author who is not a card-carrying researcher, he is also among those who rigorously urge increased research. Probably everyone would agree professionally on the need for more research, but what kind of research?

There are three areas that stand out in my mind as needing more research atttention. First, we need more attention to the environment—the contextual and situational factors—for example, Engel's (Chapter 1) scale of hierarchical systems. At the upper level, we have to think about costs. Almost every issue can be reduced to an economic and financing problem at some point. However fine our theory and elegant our teams and plans, we always run into serious cost problems. They seem insoluble. Some say that we already allocate plenty of money, but distribute it poorly. I am not sure if that is the case. Stanford Ross (1979) points out that the United States allocates less of its gross national product to social security than almost any other industrialized nation. We have the kind of leeway to develop financial support systems for older persons that many other countries such as Sweden, Holland, and Great Britain lack because they are already putting more money into social security. Also, we allocate a great deal of money to health care, but we do not spend it to the greatest advantage of the elderly. There is room for research and theoretical development as to what our nation as a whole can do to improve this larger situation in which the doctor-patient relationship takes place.

Political action by the aged is a very important issue, as our legislators have noticed. The State of Ohio allocated money to each of its seven medical schools to create offices of geriatric medicine, a very clear message from the voters (through the legislature) that something must be done about the needs of older people. The legislators are aware that a large number of older people vote more consistently than younger people do. The political issue around the care of the aged now is becoming articulated. Professionals may be able to participate constructively and help guide this movement in a useful direction. The financing pattern determines the kinds of relationships with patients that are possible.

Demographic change has been mentioned frequently. Although we all know the figures, I am not sure that we have looked thoroughly at all the implications of this demographic change. Rosow (Chapter 12) talked about cultural change and what it implies. What about some of the other changes that accompany the unprecedented predominance of older people in our society, such as the change in women's status? What wili this change do to the friends and family upon whom we depend so heavily at the present time? What about changes in the structure of the family? Who will be the future caretakers? We may not have as many immigrants as we used to, but we do have in-migrants to urban areas, who have come in very large numbers in the last 30 or 40 years. We have unrecognized immigrants coming across the Mexican border. The changing demographic character of our population has implications for the elderly. There is a change in the health-care team. Estes (Chapter 11) covers that topic beautifully.

The pharmacist is one member of the health-care team who has not been otherwise mentioned. A new law in California authorizes pharmacists to write drug prescriptions for nursing home patients. The pharmacist has suddenly become an important member of the health-care team. How does he fit in?

We also do not know enough about health-services research. We need macroeconomic and microeconomic studies and studies of how our nursing homes and health-care teams operate. Goss (Chapter 13) reminds us that we need more empirical data on these topics.

The second general area in which we need more research is health and health maintenance. There is much to be said for the salutogenic model. We should take special note of Shanas' (Chapter 3) finding that 50 percent of older people reported themselves as being well, and yet 25 percent of them saw a doctor within the previous month. Something is going on here: there is a changing definition of illness or health among older people, and we need to learn more about it. We know too little about the distinctions among disease, diagnosis, disability, and illness. They are all different, but the terms are often used interchangeably. In looking at populations of older people, we must be more precise then we have been about these distinctions. How does the patient get into the health-care system?

It is easy to forget that health care usually begins with what Freidson (1961) calls the lay referral system. We need to pay attention to interfaces, to how people get into the health-care system and move out of it. For example, not everyone who goes into a nursing home dies there. Interfaces between systems are very important at the biochemical level, and they are obviously also important at the social level. We need a dynamic model; even the triads that Rosow (Chaper 12) describes change. The family changes, the structure and composition of the family changes, and people move into and out of the house. Their conception of who belongs to the family changes. The fact that family members can function as both caregivers and barriers to care reminds us that the fact that an older person has family and friends, often lumped together as "human resources," does not necessarily mean that they are working toward his or her good.

One final area where more research is needed is more acquisition of empirical data rather than thinking primarily in terms of large-scale models, systems, and interactional models. The testing of those models against reality is of the utmost importance. We need observational studies. Technologies are available that have not been adequately used. Studies of doctor-patient interaction need to be made using videotape recordings. This technique is being used in teaching family medicine, but it has not been exploited enough for its research potential. Videotape techniques enable us to observe directly actual interaction and exchange between the doctor and patient, particularly the more complicated situations, and find out how reality fits our models. We need more case studies, studies of individuals, studies of teams, and studies of nursing homes.

In conclusion, one can hope that there will be later volumes dealing with this topic, in which more empirical data will be available for use and where tests of some intriguing models discussed by the authors of this book may be presented. Until that time, may this first collection of essays on the doctor-patient relationship and aging stimulate theory, research, and practice.

16

Research Needs in Understanding the Physician–Older Patient Relationship

M. POWELL LAWTON, Ph.D

Every chapter in this book may be looked upon as a compendium of needed research. One is struck with the richness of ideas generated by this general topic and by the intense motivation to produce knowledge that can be applied to the interchange between physician and older patient. At the same time, the conclusion is thrust upon us starkly that a great deal of the hard data comes from research on the general adult population and not with the older patient explicitly. It may well be that older people conform to the same rules that everyone else does in most instances. But we cannot be sure until the assertion has been tested. Beyond this general point that much earlier work requires replication with the aged, however, a number of more specific research needs are evident.

Discussion of these needs may best be organized in terms that bear some resemblence to the systems model articulated by Engel, which is to one extent or another also implicit in the views of many contributors. Major components of the system are the patient, the physician, the microcontext, and the macrocontext. If all of these are "input" (to use a rather tired term), we must look for ultimate results ("output"), which are, first, the patient's health and, second, the patient's sense of satisfaction in the sector of life relating to health care. This leaves us with "process," the large middle that includes the patient-physician interaction, many aspects of physician behavior, quality-of-care indicators, and patient behavior.

Many aspects of process are often viewed as ultimate criteria, but largely by default because of the major problems involved in assessing the direct effect on patients. Thus, we need to reemphasize the fact that much of what may be subsumed under "the patient-physician relationship" represents an outcome for some purposes, but ideally it should then serve as an independent variable whose effect on the ultimate criterion, patient welfare, can be studied. But let us now examine these components separately, realizing that, like every good system, one blends into another.

The Patient

As a psychologist, in assessing research needs I naturally would look particularly toward intrapersonal processes; as an environmental psychologist, I naturally would look toward the interface between environmental events and intrapersonal processes. The material relevant to these issues in the literature is minimal, forcing the realization that disparate traditions will require some new research links if we are to understand more about how personality and the external world interact in determining health attitudes, behavior, and affective outcomes.

Several authors have called attention to the crucial differences between the way acute illness and chronic illness are handled by the health-care system and responded to by individual physicians. Nonetheless, it is a matter of some concern that so little knowledge exists regarding the effect of type of illness or the response of the physician or the larger system on the individual. Weiss and the rest of us wonder what the stimulus value of the label "senile dementia" may be in the illness career of the older person. Some of Rosow's (Chapter 12) issues may be looked upon as characteristics of the patient that have major potential for determining the course of treatment and outcome.

Education is certainly one such characteristic, as are experience with the health bureaucracy and socialization to the ideology of consumerism. The patient's expectations enter strongly into the dynamics of Rosow's triads, along with intrapersonal factors like needs for technical competence and personalized respect as articulated by Marshall (Chapter 9). Shanas, Weiss, Breslau, and Goss (Chapters 3, 8, 10, and 13) repeatedly refer to the patient's attribution of difficulties to old age as a means of avoiding a perhaps more-demanding problem-solving stance. But, perhaps an attempt should be made to link such intrapersonal processes to intermediate or ultimate outcomes.

Amid the general neglect of the physician-patient relationship among the elderly, a very long time ago Alvin Goldfarb (1962) had some interesting things to say about psychotherapy with the aged, which Weiss has elaborated in his chapter. Goldfarb suggested that since many forces in the personal and social situations of aging impel persons toward greater dependence on others, the psychotherapist should accept this need in the patient—indeed, not only accept, but actively encourage the building of a dependency relationship. This was quite a radical thought coming in the tradition of twentieth-century American therapeutic philosophies of growth, self-actualization, "escape to freedom," and so on. Goldfarb felt that the dependencies of old age were a realistic consequence of both biological decline and the social deprivations of aging in our society, and thus legitimate to satisfy. He saw much unnecesary tension being heaped on the elderly expressly because the wider society rejected dependency-need satisfaction as a personal goal, not discriminating between early and middle adulthood, where the negative value judgment regarding dependency was perhaps more justified, and late life, where support from others was a much more pervasive requirement.

Goldfarb's view was not naïvely unidimensional, however. In Maslovian fashion, he saw the comfort derived from having one's dependency needs met by an appropriate supporter (i.e., the physician) as having a liberating effect, so that higher-order needs could then become satisfied. How one went beyond the stage of patient-physician dependency was not specified in detail. Nonetheless, the strong message came through that lack of self-sufficiency was the norm for the aged, and the therapist had better be willing to share some of his or her strengths with the patient.

This view thus articulates a theoretical rationale for the traditional authority role of the physician vis-à-vis the patient. The dynamics of the interaction apply equally well to both psychiatric and other forms of medical treatment.

We have heard a great deal about how the traditional authority pattern may have altered in the face of structural changes in the macroenvironment of health care, the growth of prevention as a goal, and the evolution of consumerism. Evidence is also at hand suggesting a lag in the effect of these changes among today's cohort of elderly (Haug & Lavin, 1978; Pope, 1978). However, I am not aware of any attempt to explore Goldfarb's basic hypothesis on an individual psychological level.

The Goldfarb view is strongly at variance with other conclusions that might be drawn from several streams of research in personality and social psychology. In the most general terms, this research demonstrates that a variety of favorable outcomes is associated with autonomous, as contrasted with dependent, behavior. One such stream is Rotter's (1966) social learning theory, which is concerned with how the individual learns to cope with social situations and environmental events. In his terms, "locus of control" represents the learned expectancy that an individual develops regarding the relative significance of self versus the external world as determinants of behavior. The "external" individual sees reinforcement of his or her behavior as coming from the actions of others, from external events, chance, and so on. The "internal" individual sees wishes, needs, and behavior as determined within the self. Such generalized expectancies are particularly potent as determinants of behavior when the total context is relatively lacking in clear cues as to how one should behave.

The analogy to the health-treatment situation is obvious. As Bloom and Speedling note (Chapter 14), ambiguity is great, given the disparity of knowledge between physician and patient, problems in communication, and the high level of anxiety in the patient that tends to mask cognitive processes based more on the realities of the situation than on the generalized expectancy.

In any case, the literature indicates that a variety of indicators of psychological health are associated with internality (Kuypers, 1972), and some treatment outcomes may vary with the match between degree of internality and the extent to which the environment facilitates self-determination (Reid, Haas, & Hawkings, 1977). Two possible questions may be thus posed: First, since the generalized expectancy presumably remains modifiable by further learning, can the physician-patient relationship be used as the vehicle for assisting those older people who are more external to develop further in the direction of the more favorable internal side? Second, does the physician's behavior that encourages dependency have a particularly strong negative impact on "internals?"

Although developing from a different, more cognitive, tradition, the phenomenon of learned helplessness is clearly related to the internal-external control concept. Seligman suggests that the ability to solve problems or cope with stressful situations is inhibited by previous exposure to other situations in which the subject endures stress and finds that *no* effort of his or her own can terminate the stress (Seligman, 1975). The original formulation of the theory came in relation to the study of dogs exposed to electric shock while harnessed in place, but a growing body of later research has confirmed these general conclusions among humans (Abramson, Seligman, & Teasdale, 1977).

In addition to inhibiting problem solution and the motivation to seek solutions, the perception that one's own efforts have no effect leads to the cognition that one is a failure, and ultimately to depression. Again, it is clear that, at least by analogy, the creation of a social situation—medical treatment in which the link between individual behavior and outcome is clouded by the heavy overlay of physical authority—is likely to reinforce feelings of helplessness and, conceivably, to lead to depression.

This situation seems possible to investigate either experimentally (by prescribing contrasting roles for a physician to play in a controlled situation) or naturalistically (by measuring authority behavior on the part of the physician and relating it to patient outcomes).

My discussion thus far has avoided the issue of the stability of externality or learned helplessness and the related issue of whether change is best achieved by applying effort to the older individual or to the external environment, in other words, the physician or the health-care context. A good case can be made on rational grounds that a generalized expectancy can become so overlearned over a lifetime as to act like an enduring personality "trait" rather than a situationally determined behavior. One may also ask whether there is not a moderate range where externality or helplessness (read "need for dependence") is a normally varying personality style or preference, without necessarily being pathological or leading to depression. And as Bloom and Speedling suggest, another determinant of the appropriateness of the authority stance is the extent of disablement involved.

One would thus wish to add the element of lifelong need or preference regarding autonomy versus dependence to the prediction equation. By doing so, we avoid the naïveté of the question, "Is gratified dependency or autonomy better for the older person in the doctor-patient relationship?" Rather, the question that should be researched is that of determining whether there are differential effects of dependence or autonomy, depending on whether one prefers the dependent or the ascendent role. Congruence between the individual and the external context is thus seen as more important than individual need or context alone (Kahana, in press; Lawton & Nahemow, 1973).

The concept of "a dependent relationship" will surely turn out to be more complex than it appears on the surface. For example, some possible aspects of physician behavior that contribute to dependency may include the physician's hoarding of information, his need to nurture, to wield power, and so on, each of which must be examined in terms of its place in the total constellation. Of course, the many structural factors that have been explored in such depth in many of these chapters also belong in the predictive model.

Finally, the research on sick role reviewed by Coe (Chapter 2) and on illness definition and attribution by Kart (Chapter 7) demonstrates the fact that there is still much more to learn about age differences in the way one's own views and society's views (or what goes on outside one's own somatopsyche) are perceived and integrated.

The Physician

Marshall (Chapter 9) suggests that research attempting to explain physician behavior in terms of physician characteristics has yielded meager results. He concludes that we ought better to seek explanations in the organization of health care. It would seem that before individual physician characteristics are thrown out, however, we ought to look more closely at the physician's attitudes toward the older patient and at personal factors underlying these attitudes. Ageism in the medical world has been amply noted by many writers in this book and in many other contexts. However, it seems to me that the store of solid research in this area is miniscule. For one thing, few of us see ourselves as ageists or are likely to characterize ourselves that way publicly. Thus, most of the unsubtle attitude research now in hand should, I feel, be written off as reflecting such matters as response styles, rather than true interpersonal response tendencies. We need more in-depth and open-ended inquiry within the framework of both clinical psychology and ethnography to be able to sort out the structural and the psychological bases for negative factors in the physician-patient relationship.

One interesting line of research is that dealing with the victim as a social stimulus. Lerner, Miller, and Holmes (1976) have suggested that one of the "rules" used by people to structure the external world is that the consequences of behavior are those "deserved" by the behaver—the "just world" ideology. Since the idea of the "innocent victim" is dissonant with such cognitive structure, the way to restore balance is to derogate the victim. Wortman and Dunkel-Shetter (1979) have suggested that this is one factor explaining the medical team's frequent rejection of the cancer patient; it may well apply to the older patient with all kinds of health problems, if age is seen as a state of victimization. Breslau (Chapter 10) commented that blaming the victim provides a very convenient way out of the sense of helplessness felt by the health professional when dealing with a person whose condition is viewed as inevitably proceeding downhill. It would seem that applying research using the just-world paradigm to physician behavior might well net us useful information.

Several authors are less pessimistic than Marshall about the prospects for change in treatment coming from change in one intraphysician characteristic: their reservoir of relevant knowledge about aging patients. Williams and Maddox (Chapters 4 and 6) in particular suggest that the acquisition of knowledge is the best defense for the physician against the anxiety of felt helplessness and inability to perform the curative task. In light of a study by Brubaker and Baresi (1979) that failed to support the knowledge-gives-better-treatment hypothesis, we clearly need further reseach on this issue explicitly with the physician as a subject and the aged person as the patient. And the research should concern itself with behavioral outcomes, not simply with attitudes.

Patient-Physician

Virtually every contributor in one way or another has cautioned us against a static view of processes mediating the patient-physician relationship. "Power," "authority," "dependency" and so on sound static, and if we are not careful, our own thinking can go this way. We have been properly reminded of the dynamic quality, the negotiation and renegotiation, that goes on constantly. Clearly, most topics discussed above under the categories of "patient" and "physician" in fact belong already to neither one or the other but are themselves processes.

However, for heuristic purposes, some processes seem more easily discussed as transactions. First and most obvious among these is communication between patient and physician. This topic has been mentioned in general terms by several authors. Without question we need to know a great deal about how both knowledge and affect are transmitted between these two actors. Such research is needed on the fine details of conversational interchange: How is information imparted by the physician heard, responded to, stored, and behaved toward by the patient? To what extent are concerns of the patient responded to by the physician, with what affect, and with what connotative meaning? These are essential elements required for the understanding of compliance behavior. A great deal has been learned about psychotherapy by the painstaking study of audio- or video-taped transactions. This has been totally absent from the scene of the aging patient in the consultation room.

Again, we are indebted to Marshall for calling our attention to a very important distinction to be made about aspects of treatment that go beyond the basic ingredient of the technical competence sought by the patient from the physician. It is very worthwhile to be reminded of the importance accorded "personalized respect" as a context for all physician care. To stop for a moment on this point, we could use more research that attempts to define the optimal *mix* of perceived competence and perceived respect for different types of treatment situations or illnesses.

Even more important, Marshall has sharply distinguished "personalized respect" from total psychosocial care; the latter is by no mean always appropriate; in fact, it may be perceived by the patient as intrusive. It is all too easy in a caregiving atmosphere espousing concern for the patient in total context to take the inappropriate further step of assuming that the caregiver should become an actor in the wider context. Breslau's case illustration and discussion is clearly in the biopsychosocial mold, but his call is for recognition and understanding by the physician, not for the assumption of a role larger than that wished by the patient. Research can be looked to for clarification of the relationship between degree of disability, on the one hand, and the extent to which professional roles ought to extend beyond their usual technical boundaries, on the other hand.

Contexts of Care

Without lingering over knotty problems of definition faced by environmental psychologists in imposing a taxonomy onto the world "out there," let us define the microenvironment for our purpose in both human and physical terms, that is, people in face-to-face relations with the patient or physician and the physical context in which such meetings occur: home, office, hospital, nursing home.

"Personal space" (Sommer, 1969), was not mentioned by any contributor. Personal space can be viewed as a bubble of varying size surrounding the individual which is to some extent home territory and within which the behaviors of others may take on meanings different from those that they might have if conducted at a different distance. The nursing profession has rightly become concerned with the effect of physical distance from the patient, gestures, body contact, eye contact, voice volume, and so on. These issues remain relatively unexplored in the patient-physician relationship.

Rosow's detailed consideration of some of the things that can occur when another party, a family member, enters the microenvironment constitutes an excellent call for research, which could be performed both naturalistically and experimentally. We should undoubtedly view the family as a component of the total system and concern ourselves with understanding how the anxieties, the expectations, the competing demands, and the role reversals of family members codetermine outcomes of the patient-physician transaction. My colleague Elaine Brody is conducting research currently with the evocative title "Women in the Middle." It is very clear that changes in the macrosocial structure such as gender roles need to be taken into account in understanding and using the expertise of younger family members in treatment.

Goss's concern over the varieties of control inherent in the locus of treatment brings to mind research in the theoretical mold of learned helplessness that deals with one of the extreme situations of autonomy loss: the institution for the elderly. Schulz (1976) found positive health and behavioral outcomes to follow from increasing the predictability of a nursing home environment, predictability being seen as one aspect of autonomy. Other work by Schulz and Hanusa (1979) and by Langer and Rodin (1976) has shown similar positive effects when actual opportunities to make choices were provided for nursing-home residents.

Goss has identified the radically different levels of control inherent in the treatment situation, depending on whether it is a clinic, a hospital, or a nursing home. Her thoughts offer a very clear view of research needed to document the difference and to explore the consequences of changing amount of control. The further enlargement of areas for control, of course, involves the formidable task of changing the complex authority-laden structure of the institutional care system. But the hints given at the possible far-reaching effects of enhancing autonomy in relatively small ways should encourage the application of similar techniques to the physician-patient relationship.

The mainstream of environmental psychology (Proshansky, Ittelson, & Rivlin, 1976; Lawton, 1980) has been very much concerned about the influence of the physical environment on the behavior that occurs in it. The physician's office, so far as I know, has been subjected to only limited research. One might wish to know more about how access (distance, local traffic conditions, transportation systems, parking, physical security, barriers, and pathways in and outside the office) affects the maintenance of the relationship. Privacy and the affective connotations of decor are other aspects of the microenvironment warranting our attention.

The hospital and the nursing home have, in fact, had considerable attention paid them by environmental researchers thus far, but very little with explicit attention to where the patient-physician transaction occurs. Such a research look might well show that the majority of these transactions in nursing homes occur via the patient's chart rather than face-to-face. But it is a matter for some concern that so many occasions for institution-based contact occur in public, with the physician walking by, with his eyes elsewhere, and at times that are unpredictable by the patient. A baseline of purely ecological, descriptive information on where, when, and how contact occurs in institutions would be most helpful.

As a number of authors have made clear, the physician is very frequently not a free agent in determining the conditions under which the relationship with the aged patient occurs. Too often, regulations prescribe, reimbursement limits, and the employment market channels; it becomes easy to feel like a pawn in the face of institutional and social forces. Conceptualizations regarding the macroenvironment such as those of Bloom and Speedling and provocative conclusions on the relative impact of structural versus personal causes such as those offered by Marshall, should offer motivation for researchers to pursue the interface between the individual patient or physician and these distal forces. We must remember that the macroenvironment does not act directly upon the individual in the manner of the sun or air quality. It must be perceived, organized into comprehensible chunks, interpreted, and acted upon by individuals. In the process, they impose their idiosyncratic interpretations, comply to a greater or lesser extent, and even alter the macroenvironment. Therefore, it behooves us to look further into the way that professionals and patients structure the medical-care environment. We may well find that there are consistent ways of structuring the health-care context (for example, an "ideology of impotence" or a "work-all-the angles" approach) that vary across individual physicians and add independent variance to the prediction of the outcome of the transaction with the patient.

The Outcome: What Is It?

Of all the research priorities that might be noted, top position should be given to the continuing problem of defining a criterion by which the quality of care might be judged. Part of the task would be to pare down the size of the sector of patient well-being wherein a significant effect might be expected. Another part would be to define more explicitly which component of the doctor-patient relationship might be expected to show an impact. Perhaps we should exclude criteria such as the reversal of nervous system pathology. On the other hand, we probably should include functional performance, such as ambulation or even remembering how to get to the physician's office.

It should be clear that very little research has selected an appropriate patient-illness criterion and successfully related it to behavior or attitudes stemming from the patient-physician relationship. Thus, Goss is correct in underlining the importance of patient satisfaction as an alternative or complementary indicator of outcome. However, we must also be deeply suspicious of head-on attempts to measure in any absolute sense the degree of satisfaction experienced by older people toward any aspect of their current situation (Campbell, Converse, & Rodgers, 1976; Carp, 1975; Lawton, 1979). There are many factors operating in concert that have a leveling effect on the overt critical ability of the elderly. It would be wiser to use consumer-survey approaches to compare contrasting objects (e.g., older patients exposed to two approaches to the relationship) or to compare subgroups (e.g., urban versus small-town patients) rather than to interpret the absolute percentages of those who approve a procedure as indicative of its true evaluation.

Thus, in conclusion, it may pay us to work backward through the system from the criterion problem. If we can define a few usable criteria, then the elements of the patient-physician process—that "large middle" referred to earlier—may receive some validation and themselves become usable proxy indicators of quality. As it is now, we are on very uncertain ground in asserting that process indicators such as positive attitudes toward the elderly or length of time spent with patients are by definition positive quality indicators.

REFERENCES
AND BIBLIOGRAPHY

References and Bibliography

Abdellah, F. G. "A Nationwide Study to Evaluate the Care of Patients in Nursing Homes." *Public Health Reports* 92:30–32, 1977.

Abramson, L. Y., Seligman, M. E., and Teasdale, J. D. "Learned Helplessness in Humans: Critique and Reformulation." *Psychological Bulletin*, 84:838–851, 1977.

Alonzo, A. A. "The Aged and Acute Illness Behavior." Paper presented at meetings of the Gerontological Society, San Francisco, 1977.

Andersen, R., Anderson, O. W., and Smedby, B. "Perception of and Response to Symptoms of Illness in Sweden and the U.S." *Medical Care* 6:18–30, 1968.

Andersen, R., Kravitz, J., and Anderson, O. W. "The Public's View of the Crisis in Medical Care: An Impetus for Changing Delivery Systems?" *Economic and Business Bulletin* 24 (fall): 44–52, 1971.

Anderson, F. "The Role of the Physician." In *Care of the Elderly: Meeting the Challenge of Dependency*, pp. 169–175. Ed. by A. N. Exton-Smith and J. G. Evans. New York: Academic Press, 1977.

Antonovsky, A. *Health, Stress, and Coping.* San Francisco: Jossey-Bass, 1979.

Arluke, A., Kennedy, L., and Kessler, R. C. "Re-Examining the Sick Role Concept: An Empirical Assessment." *Journal of Health and Social Behavior* 20:30–36, 1979.

Artiss, K., and Levine, A. "Doctor-Patient Relationship in Severe Illness." *New England Journal of Medicine* 288:1210–1214, 1973.

Auerbach, M., Gordon, D., Ullman, A., and Weisel, M. "Health Care in a Selected Urban Elderly Population—Utilization Patterns and Perceived Needs." *Gerontologist*, 17 (Aug.):341-346, 1977.

Balint, M. *The Doctor, His Patient and the Illness.* rev. ed. New York: International Universities Press, 1972.

Baric, L. "Recognition of the At-Risk Role: A Means to Influence Health Behavior." *International Journal of Health Education* 12:24–34, 1969.

Barker, R., Wright, B. A., and Gonick, M. R. *Adjustment to Physical Handicap and Illness: A Survey of the SocialPsychology of Physique and Disability.* New York: Social Science Research Council, 1946.

Bates, B. "Doctor and Nurse: Changing Roles and Relations." *New England Journal of Medicine* 283 (July):129–134, 1970.

Becker, H. S., and Strauss, A. L. "Careers, Personality and Adult Socialization." *American Journal of Sociology* 62 (November):253–263, 1956.

Benedict, R. "Continuities and Discontinuities in Cultural Conditioning." *Psychiatry* 1:161–167, 1938.

Bengston, V. L., and Haber, D. A. "Sociological Approaches to Aging." In *Aging: Scientific Perspectives and Social Issues*, pp. 70–91. Ed. by D. Woodruf and J. Birren. New York: Van Nostrand, 1975.

Ben-Sira, Z. "The Function of the Professional's Affective Behavior in Client Satisfaction: A Revised Approach to Social Interaction Theory." *Journal of Health and Social Behavior* 17:3–11, 1976.

Bercanovic, E. "Lay Conceptions of the Sick Role." *Social Forces* 51:63–64, 1972.

Bias, R. R., and Crawford, S. "OARS Training Program in Techniques of Adult Day Care Assessment." *Advances in Research* 3:2, 1979.

Bloom, S. W. *The Doctor and His Patient: A Sociological Interpretation*. New York: The Free Press, 1965.

Bloom, S. W., and Summey, P. "Models of the Doctor-Patient Relationship: A History of the Social System Concept." In *The Doctor-Patient Relationship in the Changing Health Scene*, pp. 17–41. Ed. by E. B. Gallagher. Washington, D.C.: DHEW Pub. No. 78–183, 1978.

Bloom, S. W., and Wilson, R. N. "Patient-Practitioner Relationships." In *Handbook of Medical Sociology*, third ed. pp. 275–296. Ed. by H. E. Freeman, L. Levine, and L. G. Reeder. Englewood Cliffs, N.J.: Prentice-Hall, 1979.

Bloor, M. J., and Horobin, G. W. "Conflict and Conflict Resolution in Doctor-Patient Interactions." In *Sociology of Medical Practice*, pp. 271–284. Ed. by A. Mead and C. Cox. London: Collier-Macmillan, 1975.

Bogdonoff, M. D. "The Physicians' Expectations and Medical Care for the Elderly." *The Gerontologist*, 10 (Spring):9–12, 1970.

Boreham, P., and Gibson, D. "The Informative Process in Private Medical Consultations: A Preliminary Investigation." *Social Science and Medicine* 12:409–416, 1978.

Breytspraak, L. M. "The Doctor-Patient Relationship and the Older Patient: A Critical Review of the Issues." Paper presented at annual meeting of the Gerontological Society, Washington, D.C.,1979.

———. "Medical Texts as Sources of Physician Attitudes Toward the Geriatric Patient." Paper presented at annual meeting of the Gerontological Society, Dallas, Texas, 1978.

Brickner, P., Duque, T., Kaufman, A., Sarg, M., Jahre, J., Maturlo, S., and Janeski, J. "The Homebound Aged: A Medically Unreached Group." *Annals of Internal Medicine*, 82 (Jan.):1–6, 1975.

Brook, R. H., and Williams, K. N. "Quality of Health Care for the Disadvantaged." *Journal of Community Health*, 1(Winter):132–136, 1975.

Brown, N. K., and Donovan, J. T. "Nontreatment of Fever in Extended-Care Facilities." *The New England Journal of Medicine*, 300(May):1246–1250, 1979.

Brubaker, T. H., and Barresi, C. M. "Social Workers' Levels of Knowledge about Old Age and Perceptions of Service Delivery to the Elderly." *Research on Aging* 1:213–232, 1979.

Butler, R. "The Doctor and the Aged Patient." In *The Geriatric Patient*, pp. 199–206. Ed. by William Reichel. New York: HP Publishing, 1978.

————. *Why Survive? Being Old in America*. New York: Harper and Row, 1975.

Butler, R., and Lewis, M. *Aging and Mental Health*. St. Louis: Mosby, 1973.

Callahan, D. "Health and Society: Some Ethical Imperatives." *Daedalus*, 106:23–34, 1977.

Campbell, A., Converse, P. E., and Rodgers, W. L. *The Quality of American Life: Perceptions, Evaluations, and Satisfactions*. New York: Russell Sage, 1976.

Carp, F. M. "Ego Defense or Cognitive Consistency Effects of Environmental Evaluation." *Journal of Gerontology*, 30:707–716, 1975.

Cartwright, A. "Prescribing and the Relationship Between Patients and Doctors." In *Social Aspects of the Medical Use of Pyschotropic Drugs*, pp. 63–74. Ed. by R. Copperstock. Toronto: Alcoholism and Drug Addiction Research Foundation of Ontario, 1974.

————. *Patients and Their Doctors: A Study of General Practice*. London: Routledge and Kegan Paul, 1967.

Cartwright, L. K. "Sources and Effects of Stress in Health Careers." In *Health Psychology—A Handbook*, pp. 419–445. Ed. by G. C. Stone, F. Cohen, N. E. Adler, and associates. San Francisco: Jossey-Bass, 1979.

Caterinicchio, R. P. "Testing Plausible Path Models of Interpersonal Trust in Patient-Physician Treatment Relationships." *Social Science and Medicine* 13:89–99, 1979.

Cavan, R. S. "Self and Role in Adjustment During Old Age." In *Gerontology: A Book of Readings*, pp. 122–130. Ed. by C. B. Vedder. Springfield, Ill: Thomas, 1971.

Child, Irvin L. "Socialization." In *The Handbook of Social Psychology*, first ed., pp. 655–692. Ed. by Gardner Lindzey. Reading, Mass.: Addison-Wesley, 1954.

Clayton, P. "The Clinical Morbidity of the First Year of Bereavement: A Review." *Comprehensive Psychiatry* 14:151–157, 1973.

Coe, R.M. *Sociology of Medicine*. New York: McGraw-Hill, 1970.

Coe, R. M., and Brehm, H. P. "Preventive Health Services and Physician Error." *Social Science and Medicine* 7:303–305, 1973.

————. *Preventive Health Care for Adults: A Study of Medical Practice*. New Haven, Conn.: College and University Press, 1972.

Coe, R. M., Pepper, M., and Mattis, M. "The 'New' Medical Student: Another View." *Journal of Medical Education* 52 (Feb.):89–98, 1977.

Coe, R. M., and Peterson, W. A. *The Impact of Medicare in Selected Communities*. Washington, D.C.: Institute for Community Studies, Final Report SSA#71 #3400, 1973.

Coe, R. M., and Wessen, A. F. "Social-Psychological Factors Influencing the Use of Community Health Resources." *American Journal of Public Health* 55:1024–1031, 1965.

Cohen, G. "Approach to the Geriatric Patient." *Medical Clinics of North America*, 61 (July):855–866, 1977.

Collins, R. *Conflict Sociology: Toward an Explanatory Science*. New York: Academic Press, 1975.

Columbia University, School of Public Health and Administration. *The Quantity, Quality and Costs of Medical and Hospital Care Secured by a Sample of Team-*

ster Families in the New York Area. New York: Columbia University, 1962.

Congalton, A. "Public Evaluation of Medical Care." *Medical Journal of Australia* 24:1165–1171, 1969.

Coser, L. A. "Two Methods in Search of a Substance." In *The Uses of Controversy in Sociology,* pp. 329-341. Ed. by L. A. Coser and O. N. Larsen. New York: Free Press, 1976.

Coser, L. A., and Larsen, O. N. (eds.). *The Uses of Controversy in Sociology.* New York: Free Press, 1976.

Crane, D. *The Sanctity of Social Life: Physicians' Treatment of Critically Ill Patients.* New York: Russell Sage Foundation, 1975.

Current Population Report. Series 25, No. 870, Table 1. Washington, D.C.: Current Population Reports, 1980.

Cyrus-Lutz, C., and Gaitz, C. "Psychiatrists' Attitudes Toward the Aged and Aging." *The Gerontologist* 12:163–167, 1972.

Danziger, S. K. "The Uses of Expertise in Doctor-Patient Encounters During Pregnancy." *Social Science and Medicine* 12 (Sept.):359–367, 1978.

Davis, M. S. "Variation in Patients' Compliance with Doctors' Orders: Medical Practice and the Doctor-Patient Interaction." *Psychiatry and Medicine* 2:31–54, 1971.

———. "Attitudinal and Behavioral Aspects of the Doctor-Patient Relationship as Expressed and Exhibited by Medical Students and Their Mentors." *Journal of Medical Education* 43:337–342, 1968.

Davis, M. S., and Eichorn, R. L. "Compliance with Medical Regimens: A Panel Study." *Journal of Health and Human Behavior* 4 (winter):240–249, 1963.

DiMatteo, M. R., Prince, L. M., and Taranta, A. "Patients' Perceptions of Physicians Behavior: Determinants of Patient Commitment to the Therapeutic Relationship." *Journal of Community Health* 4:280–290, 1979.

Donabedian, A. "The Quality of Medical Care: Methods for Assessing and Monitoring the Quality of Care for Research and Quality Assurance Programs." In *Health United States,* pp. 111–126. Washington, D.C.: DHEW Publication No. 78–1232, 1978.

———. "Measuring the Quality of Medical Care." In *Medicine in a Changing Society,* second ed. pp. 151–174. Ed. by L. Corey, S. Saltman, and M. Epstein. St. Louis: Mosby, 1977.

———. "Evaluation of the Quality of Medical Care." *Milbank Memorial Fund Quarterly* 44:166–206, 1966.

Duckworth, G., Kedward, H., Eastwood, M., Allodi, F., Woogh, C., and Meier, R. "Psychiatric Diagnosis in Toronto, New York and London." *Canadian Psychiatric Association Journal,* 21 (8):533–539, 1976.

Duke Center for the Study of Aging and Human Development. *Multidimensional Functional Assessment: The OARS Methodology,* second ed. Durham, N.C.: Duke University, 1978.

Dunnell, K., and Cartwright, A. *Medicine Takers, Prescribers, and Hoarders.* London: Routledge and Kegan Paul, 1972.

Eaton, M., and Scherger, J. "Health Team Function: Testing a Method for Improvement." *Journal of Family Practice* 6:101–107, 1978.

Ehrenreich, B., and Ehrenreich, J. *The American Health Empire: Power, Profits, and Politics.* New York: Vintage, 1970.

Eisdorfer, C. "Observations on Medical Care of the Aged." In *Foundations of Practical Gerontology*, pp. 68–76. Ed. by R. R. Boyd and C. G. Oakes. Columbia, S.C.: University of South Carolina Press, 1973.

Eisenberg, J. M. "Sociologic Influences on Decision-Making by Clinicians." *Annals of Internal Medicine* 90:957–964, 1979.

Eisenthal, S., Emery, R., Lazare, A., and Udin, H. "Adherence and the Negotiated Approach to Patienthood." *Archives of General Psychiatry* 36 (Apr.):393–398, 1979.

Ellison, D. "Work, Retirement and the Sick Role." *The Gerontologist* 8:189–192, 1968.

Elmore, J. "Physician-Patient Relationship in Geriatric Treatment." *Wisconsin Medical Journal* 67 (Feb.):117–120, 1968.

Engel, G. L. "Biomedicine's Failure to Achieve Flexnerian Standards of Education." *Journal of Medical Education* 53:387–392, 1978a.

———. "The Biopsychosocial Model and the Education of Health Professionals." *Annals of the New York Academy of Sciences* 310:169–181, 1978b.

———. "Psychologic Stress, Vasodepressor (Vasovagal) Syncope and Sudden Death." *Annals of Internal Medicine* 89:403–412, 1978c.

———. "The Care of the Patient: Art or Science?" *Johns Hopkins Medical Journal* 140:222–232, 1977a.

———. "The Need for a New Medical Model: A Challenge for Biomedicine." *Science* 196:129–136, 1977b.

———. "Sudden and Rapid Death During Psychological Stress. Folklore or Folkwisdom?" *Annals of Internal Medicine* 74:771–782, 1971.

———. "A Unified Concept of Health and Disease." *Perspectives in Biology and Medicine* 3:459–485, 1960.

Erikson, E. H. *Identity: Youth and Crisis.* New York: Norton, 1968.

———. *Childhood and Society*, second ed. New York: Norton, 1963.

———. *Identity and the Life-Cycle: Psychologial Issues.* Monograph 1. New York: International Universities Press, 1959.

Exton-Smith, A. N. "Clinical Manifestations of Functional Consequences of Aging." In *Care of the Elderly: Meeting the Challenge of Dependency*, pp. 41–53. Ed. by A. N. Exton-Smith and J. G. Evans. London: Academic Press, 1977.

Fabrega, H. "The Need for an Ethnomedical Science." *Science* 189:969–975, 1975.

Feldman, J. J. *The Dissemination of Health Information.* Chicago: Aldine, 1966.

Fleming, G. V. "Satisfaction with Medical Care." Unpublished Manuscript. Chicago: Center for Health Administration Studies, University of Chicago, n.d.

Flexner, A. *Medical Education in the United States and Canada. Report of the Carnegie Foundation on the Advancement of Teaching.* Bulletin No. 4. Boston: Updyke, 1910

Ford, A. "Distinguishing Characteristics of the Aging from a Clinical Viewpoint." *Journal of the American Geriatric Society* 16:142–148, 1968.

Ford, A. B., Liske, R. E., Ort, R.S., and Denton, J. C. *The Doctor's Perspective: Physicians View Their Patients and Practice.* Cleveland: Case Western Reserve University Press, 1967.

Fox, R. C. "The Medicalization and Demedicalization of American Society." *Daedelus* 106:9–22, 1977.

——. *Experiment Perilous.* New York: Free Press, 1959.

Freedman, J., Sears, D., and Carlsmith, J. *Social Psychology,* third ed. Englewood Cliffs: N.J.: Prentice-Hall, 1978.

Freidson, E. *Doctoring Together.* New York: Elsevier, 1975.

——. *Professional Autonomy.* New York: Atherton, 1970a.

——. *Professional Dominance.* New York: Atherton, 1970b.

——. *Profession of Medicine.* New York: Dodd Mead, 1970c.

——. *Patients' View of Medical Practice.* New York: Russell Sage Foundation, 1961.

——. "Client Control and Medical Practice." *American Journal of Sociology* 65:374–382, 1960.

Freidson, E., and Feldman, J. J. *The Public Looks at Hospital.* Health Information Foundation Research Series. No. 4, 1958.

French, J. R. P., Jr., and Raven, B. H. "The Bases of Social Power." In *Studies in Social Power,* pp. 150–167. Ed. by D. Cartwright. Ann Arbor: University of Michigan, Institute of Social Research, 1959.

Fromm, E. "The Problem of the Oedipus Complex." Paper presented at Langley Porter Neuropsychiatric Institute Staff Meeting, San Francisco, April 20, 1966.

Funkenstein, D. H. *Medical Students, Medical Schools and Society During Five Eras: Factors Affecting the Career Choices of Physicians 1958–1976.* Cambridge, Mass.: Ballinger, 1978.

Gallagher, E. B. "Lines of Reconstruction and Extension in the Parsonian Sociology of Illness." *Social Science and Medicine* 10:207–218, 1976.

——. (ed.). *The Doctor-Patient Relationship in the Changing Health Scene.* Washington, D.C.: DHEW, Pub. No. 78-183, 1978.

Geertsen, H. R., Gray, R. M., and Ward, J. R. "Patient Non-Compliance with the Context of Seeking Medical Care for Arthritis." *Journal of Chronic Disease* 26:689–698, 1973.

Gerson, E. M. "The Social Character of Illness: Deviance or Politics?" *Social Science and Medicine* 10:219–224, 1976.

Gill, D. G. "Limitations Upon Choice and Constraints Over Decision-Making in Doctor-Patient Exchanges." In *The Doctor-Patient Relationship in the Changing Health Scene,* pp. 141–153. Ed. by E. B. Gallagher. Washington, D.C.: DHEW Pub. No. 78-183, 1978.

Goldfarb, A. I. "The Psychotherapy of Elderly Patients." In *Medical and Clinical Aspects of Aging,* pp. 106–114. Ed. by H. T. Blumenthal. New York: Columbia University Press, 1962.

Goldsmith, S. B. "House Calls: Anachronism or Advent?" *Public Health Reports* 94 (July–Aug.):299–304, 1979.

Goss, M. E. W. "Organizational Goals and Quality of Medical Care: Evidence from Comparative Research on Hospitals." *Journal of Health and Social Behavior* 11:255–268, 1970.

Gottesman, L. E., and Boureston, N. C. "Why Nursing Homes Do What They

Do." *Gerontologist* 14:501–506, 1974.

Gough, H. D. "Doctors' Estimates of the Percentage of Patients Whose Problems Do Not Require Medical Attention." *Medical Education* 11:380–384, 1977.

Gruber, H. "Geriatrics-Physician Attitudes and Medical School Training." *Journal of the American Geriatric Society* 25 (Nov.):494–499, 1977.

Gustafson, E. "Dying: The Career of the Nursing Home Patient." *Journal of Health and Social Behavior* 13:226–235, 1972.

Handy, R., and Zakaria, G. "A Special Clinic for the Over 65's in a GP Surgery." *Practitioner* 219 (Sept.):365–375, 1977.

Haney, C. A. "Psychosocial Factors Involved in Medical Decision-Making." In *Psychosocial Aspects of Medical Training*, pp. 404–425. Ed. by R. H. Coombs and C. E. Vincent. Springfield, Ill.: Thomas, 1971.

Harris, Louis and Associates. *Hospital Care in America. A National Opinion Research Survey of Consumers, Government Officials, and Health Care Community Attitudes Toward Health and Hospital Care.* Nashville, Tennessee: Hospital Affiliates International, 1978.

————. *The Myth and Reality of Aging in America.* Washington, D.C.: National Council on Aging, 1975.

Haug, M. R. "Doctor-Patient Relationships and the Older Patient." *Journal of Gerontology* 34:852–860, 1979.

————. "Issues in Patient Acceptance of Physician Authority in Great Britain." In *The Doctor-Patient Relationship in the Changing Health Scene*, pp. 239–254. Ed. by E. B. Gallagher. Washington, D.C.: DHEW Pub. No. 78–183, 1978.

————. "Issues in General Practitioner Authority in the National Health Service." In *The Sociology of the National Health Service, Sociological Review Monograph 22*, pp. 23–42. Ed. by M. Stacey, University of Keele, Great Britain, 1976.

Haug, M. R., and Lavin, B. "Method of Payment for Medical Care and Public Attitudes Toward Physician Authority." *Journal of Health and Social Behavior* 19:279–291, 1978.

Haug, M. R., and Sussman, M. B. "Professional Autonomy and the Revolt of the Client." *Social Problems* 17 (Fall):153–161, 1969.

Hayes-Bautista, D. E. "Chicano Patients and Medical Practitioners: A Sociology of Knowledge Paradigm of Lay-Professional Interaction." *Social Science and Medicine* 12:83–90, 1978.

————. "Termination of the Patient-Practitioner Relationship: Divorce, Patient Style." *Journal of Health and Social Behavior* 17 (Mar.): 12–21, 1976.

Haynes, R. B., Sackett, D. L., and Taylor, W. (eds.). *Compliance in Health Care.* Baltimore: Johns Hopkins University Press, 1979.

Health PAC. *The American Health Empire.* New York: Vintage Books, 1970.

Henderson, L. J. "Physician and Patient as a Social System." *New England Journal of Medicine* 18 (May):819–823, 1935.

Hoenig, J., and Ragg, N. "The Non-Attending Psychiatric Outpatient: An Administrative Problem." *Medical Care* 4:96–100, 1966.

Hornung, C. A., and Massagli, M. "Primary Care Physicians' Affective Orientation Toward Their Patients." *Journal of Health and Social Behavior* 20 (Mar.): 61–70, 1979.

Howard, E. "The Effect of Work Experience in a Nursing Home on the Attitudes Toward Death Held by Nurse Aides." *The Gerontologist* 14 (Feb.):54–56, 1974.

Hughes, E. C. "Cycles, Turning Points, and Careers." Reprinted in E. C. Hughes, *The Sociological Eye: Selected Papers on Institutions and Race.* Chicago: The University of Chicago Press, 1971.

Hurtado, A. V., Greenlick, M. R., and Colombo, T. J. "Determinants of Medical Care Utilization: Failure to Keep Appointments." *Medical Care* 11:189–198, 1973.

Illich, I. *Medical Nemesis: The Expropriation of Health.* London: Calder and Boyars, 1975.

Institute of Medicine, National Academy of Sciences. *Aging and Medical Education.* National Academy of Sciences, Washington, D.C. (Beeson Committee Report), Sept., 1978.

Janis, I., and Rodin, J. "Attribution, Control and Decision Making: Social Psychology and Health Care." In *Health Psychology—A Handbook*, pp. 487–521. Ed. by G. C. Stone, F. Cohen, N. E. Adler, and associates. San Francisco: Jossey-Bass, 1979.

Jones, E., and Nisbett, R. *The Actor and the Observer: Divergent Perceptions of the Causes of Behavior.* Morristown, N.J.: General Learning Press, 1971.

Kahana, E. "A Congruence Model of Person-Environment Interaction." In *Aging and Environment: Theoretical Approaches.* Ed. by M. P. Lawton, P. G. Windley, and T. O. Byerts. New York: Springer Publishing Company (in press).

Kahn , R., Zarit, S., Hilbert, N., and Niederehe, G. "Memory Complaint and Impairment in the Aged." *Archives of General Psychiatry* 32:1569–1573, 1975.

Kane, R. L., Solomon, D. H., Beck, J. C., Keeler, E., and Kane, R. A. "A Game of Dwindling Numbers: Medical Manpower for the Elderly." *Rand Checklist*, 229 (June):1–2, 1980.

Karasu, T., Stein, B., and Charles, E. S. "Age Factors in Patient-Therapist Relationship." *The Journal of Nervous and Mental Disease* 167:100–104, 1979.

Kart, C. S., and Manard, B. B. "Quality of Care in Old Age Institutions." *The Gerontologist* 16:250–256, 1976.

Kart, C. S., Metress, E. S., and Metress, J. F. *Aging and Health: Biologic and Social Perspectives.* Reading, Mass.: Addison-Wesley, 1978.

Kasl, S., and Cobb, S. "Health Behavior, Illness Behavior, and Sick Role Behavior." *Archives of Environmental Health* 12:246–266, 1966.

Kassebaum, G. G., and Bauman, B. O. "Dimensions of the Sick Role in Chronic Illness." *Journal of Health and Human Behavior* 6:16–27, 1965.

Kasteler, J., Kane, R. L., Olsen, D. M., and Thetford, C. "Issues Underlying Prevalence of 'Doctor-Shopping' Behavior." *Journal of Health and Social Behavior* 17:328–339, 1976.

Kastenbaum, R. "The Reluctant Therapist." In *New Thoughts on Old Age*, pp. 139–145. Ed. by R. Kastenbaum. New York: Springer, 1964.

Kelly, J., Hanson, G., Garetz, D. and Spencer, D. "What the Family Physician Should Know About Treating Elderly Patients." *Geriatrics* 32 (Oct.):79–92, 1977.

Kisch, A. I., and Reeder, L. G. "Client Evaluation of Physician Performance."

Journal of Health and Social Behavior 10 (Mar.):51–58, 1969.

Kleinman, M. B., and Clemente, F. "Support for the Medical Profession Among the Aged." *International Journal of Health Services* 6:295–299, 1976.

Kogan, N. "Beliefs, Attitudes and Stereotypes About Old People." *Research on Aging 1:11–36, 1979.*

Koos, E. *The Health of Regionville.* New York: Columbia University Press, 1954.

Kosa, J., and Robertson, L. "The Social Aspects of Health and Illness." In *Poverty and Health*, pp. 35–68. Ed. by J. Kosa, A. Antonovsky, and I. Zola. Cambridge: Harvard University Press, 1969.

Kraus, A., and Lilienfeld, A. "Some Epidemiologic Aspects of the High Mortality Rate in the Young Widowed Group." *Journal of Chronic Diseases* 10:207–217, 1959.

Krause, E. A. *Power and Illness: The Political Sociology of Health and Medical Care.* New York: Elsevier, 1977.

Kuypers, J. A. "Internal-External Locus of Control, Ego Functioning, and Personality Characteristics in Old Age." *Gerontologist* 12:168–173, 1972.

Langer, E., and Rodin, J. "The Effects of Choice and Enhanced Personal Responsibility for the Aged." *Journal of Personality and Social Psychology*, 34:191–198, 1976.

Lasagna, L. "Aging and the Field of Medicine." In *Aging and Society Vol. 2: Aging and the Professions*, pp. 55–78. Ed. by M. W. Riley, J. W. Riley, Jr., and M. E. Johnson. New York: Russell Sage Foundation, 1969.

Laurie, W. F. "Employing the Duke OARS Methodology in Cost-Comparisons: Home Services and Institutionalization." Duke University Center for the Study of Aging and Human Development *Advances in Research* 2:2 (whole issue), 1978.

———. "The Duke OARS Methodology: Basic Research and a Practical Application." Duke University Center for the Study of Aging and Human Development *Advances in Research* 1:2 (whole issue), 1977.

Lawton, M. P. *Environment and Aging.* Monterey, Calif.: Brooks/Cole, 1980.

———. "Housing Problems of the Community-Resident Elderly." *Occasional Papers in Housing and Community Affairs*, No. 1. Washington, D.C.: U.S. Government Printing Office, 1979.

———. "Social Ecology and the Health of Older People." *American Journal of Public Health* 64:257–260, 1974.

Lawton, M.P. and Nahemow, L. "Ecology and the Aging Process." In *Psychology of Adult Development and Aging*, pp. 619–674. Ed. by C. Eisdorfer and M. P. Lawton. Washington, D.C.: American Psychological Association, 1973.

Lazare, A., Eisenthal, S., Frank, A., and Stoeckle, J. D. "Studies on a Negotiated Approach to Patienthood." In *The Doctor-Patient Relationship in the Changing Health Scene*, pp. 119–139. Ed. by E.B. Gallagher. Washington, D.C.: U.S. DHEW, 1978.

Lederer, H. "How the Sick View Their World." In *Patients, Physicians and Illness*, pp. 247–268. Ed. by E. G. Jaco. Glencoe, Ill.: The Free Press, 1958.

Lebow, J. L. "Consumer Assessments of the Quality of Medical Care." *Medical Care* 12:328–337, 1974.

Lerner, M. J., Miller, D. T., and Holmes, J. "Deserving and the Emergence of Forms of Justice." *Advances in Experimental Social Psychology.* New York: Academic Press, 1976.

Levinson, D. J. *The Seasons of a Man's Life.* New York: Knopf, 1978.

Libow, L. "Pseudo-senility: Acute and Reversible Organic Brain Syndrome." *Journal of the American Geriatric Society* 21:112–120, 1973.

Lilja, J. "How Physicians Choose Their Drugs." *Social Science and Medicine* 10 (July/Aug.):358–365, 1976.

Lindemann, E. "Symptomatology and Management of Acute Grief." *American Journal of Psychiatry* 101:141–148, 1944.

Linn, B. S., Linn, M. W., and Gurel, L. "Correlates of Prognosis: A Study of the Physician's Clinical Judgment." *Medical Care* 11:430–435, 1973.

Linn, L. S. "Factors Associated with Patient Evaluation of Health Care." *The Milbank Memorial Fund Quarterly, Health and Society* 53:531–548, 1975.

Linn, M. W., Gurel, L., and Linn, B. S. "Patient Outcome as a Measure of Quality of Nursing Home Care." *American Journal of Public Health* 67:337–342, 1977.

Lipman, A. "Role Conception and Morale of Couples in Retirement." *Journal of Gerontology* 16:267–271, 1961.

Lipman, A., and Sterne, R. S. "Aging in the United States: Assumption of a Terminal Sick Role." *Sociology and Social Research* 53:194–203, 1965.

Lowenthal, M. F., Thurnher, M., and Chiriboga, D. (eds.). *Four Stages of Life.* San Francisco: Jossey-Bass, 1975.

Lown, B., Verrier, R. L., and Rabinowitz, S. H. "Neural and Psychologic Mechanisms and the Problem of Sudden Death." *American Journal of Cardiology* 39:890–902, 1977.

Lyons, T. F., and Payne, B. C. "The Quality of Physicians' Health-Care Performance." *Journal of American Medical Association* 227:925–928, 1974.

Maddox, G. L. "Interventions and Outcomes: Notes on Designing an Experiment in Health Care." *International Journal of Epidemiology* 1:339–345, 1972.

Maddox, G. L., and Dellinger, D. C. "Assessment of Functional Status in a Program Evaluation and Resource Allocation Model." *Annals of the American Academy of Political and Social Science* 438:59–70, 1978.

Marshall, V. W. *Last Chapters: A Sociology of Aging and Dying.* Monterey, Calif.: Brooks/Cole, 1980.

———. "No Exit: A Symbolic Interactionist Perspective on Aging." *International Journal of Aging and Human Development* 9:345–358, 1978.

Marshall, V. W., and Tindale, J. A. "Notes for a Radical Gerontology." *International Journal of Aging and Human Development* 9:163–175, 1978.

Maslach, C. "The Burnt-Out Syndrome and Patient Care." In *Psychosocial Care of the Dying*, pp. 111–120. Ed. by C. Garfield. New York: McGraw-Hill, 1978.

———. "Burned Out." *Human Behavior* 5:16–22, 1976.

McFarland, D. "The Aged in the 21st Century: a Demographer's View." In *Aging Into the 21st Century*, pp. 5–22. Ed. by L. F. Jarvik. New York: Gardner Press, 1978.

McKinlay, J. B. "The Changing Political and Economic Context of the Patient-Physician Encounter." In *The Doctor-Patient Relationship in the Changing Health*

Scene, pp. 155–188. Ed. by E. B. Gallagher. Washington, D.C.: U.S. DHEW, Pub. No. 78–183, 1978.

———. "The Sick-Role—Illness and Pregnancy." *Social Science and Medicine* (6):561-572, 1972.

Mead, B. "How to Relate to the Elderly Patient." *Geriatrics* 32 (Oct.): 73–77, 1977.

Mead, M. "Towards a Human Science." *Science* 191:903–909, 1976.

Mechanic, D. *Medical Sociology,* second ed. New York: Free Press, 1978.

———. "The English National Health Service: Some Comparisons with the United States." In *Public Expectations and Health Care,* pp. 185–195. Ed. by D. Mechanic. New York: Wiley-Interscience, 1972.

———. "The Concept of Illness Behavior." *Journal of Chronic Diseases* 15:189–194, 1961.

Mendenhall, R. C., Girard, R. A., and Abrahamson, S. "A National Study of Medical and Surgical Specialities I: Background, Purpose, and Methodology." *Journal of the American Medical Association*

Miller, D. B., Lowenstein, R., and Winston, R. "Physicians' Attitudes Toward the Ill Aged and Nursing Homes." *Journal of the American Geriatrics Society* 24:498–505, 1976.

Monroe, R. T. "How Well are Older People?" *Journal of the Michigan State Medical Society* 59:748–751, 1960.

Moore, J., and Kane, W. J. "Geriatric Training in Family Medicine: The Natural History of a Developing Program." *The Journal of Family Practice* 8:79 83, 1979.

Mortimer, J. T., and Simmons, R. G. "Adult Socialization." In *Annual Review of Sociology,* 4:421–454. Palo Alto: Annual Reviews, 1978.

Mumford, E. *Interns: From Students to Physicians.* Cambridge, Mass.: Harvard University Press, 1970.

Myles, J. F. "Institutionalization and Sick Role Identification Among the Elderly." *American Sociological Review* 43:508–521, 1978.

Nathanson, C. "Illness and the Feminine Role: A Theoretical Review." *Social Science and Medicine* 9:57–62, 1975.

National Center for Health Statistics. *"Physician Visits" Volume and Interval Since Last Visit, United States—1975.* Washington, D.C.: Vital Health Statistics, Series 10, No. 128. DHEW Pub. No. (PHS) 79–1556, 1979.

———. *The National Ambulatory Medical Care Survey: 1975 Summary, United States, January–December 1975.* Washington, D.C.: Vital and Health Statistics, Series 13, No. 33. DHEW Pub. No. (PHS) 78–1784, 1978.

———. *Health United States, 1978.* Washington, D.C.: DHEW Pub. No. (PHS) 78–1232, 1978.

———. *Current Estimates from the Health Interview Survey; United States—1975.* Washington, D.C.: Vital and Health Statistics, Series 10, No. 115. DHEW Pub. No. (HRA) 77–1543, 1977.

———. *Utilization of Nursing Homes, United States: National Nursing Home Survey, August 1973–April 1974.* Washington, D.C.: Vital and Health Statistics, Series 13, No. 28. DHEW Pub. No. (HRA) 77–1779, 1977.

Navarro, V. *Medicine Under Capitalism.* New York: Prodist, 1976.

Neugarten, B. L. "Age Groups in American Society and the Rise of the Young-Old." *Annals of the American Academy of Political and Social Sciences*, 415 (Sept.):187–198, 1974.

Neugarten, B. L., Moore, J. W., and Lowe, J. C. "Age Norms, Age Constraints and Adult Socialization." In *Middle Age and Aging*, pp. 22–28. Ed. by B. L. Neugarten. Chicago: University of Chicago Press, 1968.

Nuttbrock, L., and Kosberg, J. I. "Images of the Physician and Help-Seeking Behavior of the Elderly: A Multivariate Assessment." *Journal of Gerontology* 35(2):241–248, 1980.

Osborn, R. "Social Rank and Self-Health Evaluation of Older Urban Males." *Social Science and Medicine* 7:209–218, 1973.

Page, I. H. "Social Planning and Our Medical Schools." *Science* 159:261, 1968.

Palmer, R. H., and Reilly, M. C. "Individual and Institutional Variables Which May Serve as Indicators of Quality of Medical Care." *Medical Care* 17 (July):693–717, 1979.

Parkes, C. "Effects of Bereavement on Physical and Mental Health—A Study of the Medical Records of Widows." *British Medical Journal* 2:274–279, 1964.

Parsons, T. "Epilogue." In *The Doctor-Patient Relationship in the Changing Health Scene*, pp. 445–455. Ed. by E.B. Gallagher. Washington, D.C.: DHEW Pub. No. 78–183, 1978.

———. "The Sick Role and the Role of the Physician Reconsidered." *Health and Society* 53:257–277, 1975.

———. *Social Structure and Personality*. New York: Free Press, 1965.

———. "Definitions of Health and Illness in the Light of American Values and Social Structure." In *Patients, Physicians and Illness*, pp. 165–187. Ed. by E. Jaco. Glencoe, Ill.: Free Press, 1958.

———. *The Social System*. Glencoe, Ill.: The Free Press,1951.

Pathy, M. "Clinical Presentation of Myocardial Infarction in the Elderly." *British Heart Journal* 29:190–199, 1967.

Peterson, L. L., Andrews, L. P., Spain, R. S., and Greenberg, B. G. "An Analytical Study of North Carolina General Practice. *Journal of Medical Education* 31 (Dec.):1–165, 1956.

Petroni, F. "Correlates of the Psychiatric Sick Role." *Journal of Health and Social Behavior* 13:47–54, 1972.

Pfeiffer, E. "Pharmacology of Aging." In *Health Care of the Elderly*, pp. 47–68. Ed. by G. Lesnoff-Caravaglia. New York: Human Sciences Press, 1980.

Plant, J. "Various Approaches Proposed to Assess Quality in Long-Term Care." *Hospitals* 51:93–98, 1977.

Poole, A. D., and Sanson-Fisher, R. W. "Understanding the Patient: A Neglected Aspect of Medical Education." *Social Science and Medicine* 13:37–43, 1979.

Pope, C. R. "Consumer Satisfaction in a Health Maintenance Organization." *Journal of Health and Social Behavior* 19 (Sept.):291–303, 1978.

Proshansky, H. M., Ittelson, W. H., and Rivlin, L. G. (eds). *Environmental Psychology*. New York: Holt, Rinehart, and Winston, 1976.

Reader, G. C., Pratt, L., and Mudd, M. C. "What Patients Expect from Their Doctors." *Modern Hospital* 89:88–94, 1957.

Reid, D. W., Haas, G., and Hawkings, D. "Locus of Desired Control and Positive Self-Concept of the Elderly." *Journal of Gerontology*, 32:441–450, 1977.

Reiser, S. J., Dyck, A. J., and Curran, W. J. *Ethics in Medicine: Historical Perspectives and Contemporary Concerns.* Cambridge, Mass.: MIT Press, 1977.

Reynolds, R. E., and Bice, T. W. "Attitudes of Medical Interns Toward Patients and Health Professionals." *Journal of Health and Social Behavior* 12 (Dec.):307–311, 1971.

Rezler, A. G. "Attitude Changes During Medical School: A Review of the Literature." *Journal of Medical Education* 49:1023–1030, 1974.

Riley, M. W., Foner, A., Hess, B., and Toby, M. L. "Socialization for the Middle and Later Years." In *Handbook of Socialization Theory and Research*, pp. 951–982. Ed. by D. A. Goslin. Chicago: Rand McNally, 1969.

Riley, M. W., Johnson, M., and Foner, A. (eds.). *Aging and Society: A Sociology of Age Stratification.* New York: Russell Sage, 1972.

The Robert Wood Johnson Foundation. *America's Health Care System: A Comprehensive Portrait.* Special Report, No. 1, 1978.

Robinson, D. *The Process of Becoming Ill.* London: Routledge and Kegan Paul, 1971.

Rodin, J. "Somatopsychics and Attribution." *Personality and Social Psychology Bulletin* 4:531–540, 1978.

Rosati, R., McNear, F., Starmer, F., Mittler, B., Morris, J., and Wallace, A. "A New Information System for Medical Practice." *Archives of Internal Medicine* 135:1017–1024, 1975.

Rose, A. M. "The Subculture of the Aging." In *Middle Age and Aging*, pp. 29–34. Ed. by B. L. Neugarten. Chicago: University of Chicago Press, 1968.

Rosenthal, C. J., Marshall, V. W., Macpherson, A. S., and French, S. P. *Nurses, Patients and Families: Care and Control in the Hospital.* New York: Springer, 1980.

Rosenstock, I., and Kirscht, J. "Why People Seek Health Care." In *Health Psychology*, pp. 161–188. Ed. by G. Stone, F. Cohen, and N. Adler. San Francisco: Jossey-Bass, 1979.

Ross, L., Lepper, M., and Hubbard, M. "Perserverance in Self-Perception and Social Perception: Biased Attributional Processes in the Debriefing Paradigm." *Journal of Personality and Social Psychology* 32:880–892, 1975.

Ross, S. "Social Security: A Worldwide Issue." *Social Security Bulletin* 42 (Aug.):3–10, 1979.

Roth, J. "Staff and Client Control Strategies in Urban Hospital Emergency Services." *Urban Life and Culture* 1 (Apr.):39–60, 1972.

———. *Timetables.* Indianapolis: Bobbs-Merrill, 1963.

Rotter, J. B. "Generalized Expectancies for Internal Versus External Control of Reinforcement." *Psychological Monographs*, 80:1 (whole No. 609), 1966.

Rubin, I. M., Plovnick, M. S., Fry, R. E. *Improving the Coordination of Care: A Program of Health Team Development.* Cambridge, Mass.: Ballinger, 1975.

Ryan, W. *Blaming the Victim.* New York: Vintage, 1971.

Schouten, J. "Important Factors in the Examination and Care of Old Patients." *Journal of the American Geriatrics Society* 23:180–183, 1975.

Schulz, R. "Effects of Control and Predictability on the Physical and Psychological Well-being of the Institutionalized Aged." *Journal of Personality and Social Psychology* 33:563–573, 1976.

Schulz, R., and Hanusa, B. H. "Environmental Influences on the Effectiveness of Control and Competence-enhancing Interventions." In *Choice and Perceived Control*, pp. 315–337. Ed. by R. A. Monty and L. C. Pearlmutter. New York: Lawrence Erlebaum Associates, 1979.

Schwartz, D., Henley, B., and Zeitz, L. *The Elderly Ambulatory Patient*. New York: Macmillan, 1964.

Segall, A. "The Sick Role Concept: Understanding Illness Behavior." *Journal of Health and Social Behavior* 17:163–170, 1976a.

———."Sociocultural Variations in Sick Role Behavioral Expectations." *Social Science and Medicine* 10:47–51, 1976b.

Seligman, M. E. *Helplessness: On Depression, Development and Death*. San Francisco: Freeman, 1975.

Shanas, E. "The Status of Health Care for the Elderly." In *Health Care of the Elderly*, pp. 167–176. Ed. by G. Lesnoff-Caravaglia. New York: Human Sciences Press, 1980.

———. *Final Report. National Survey of the Aged. A Report to the Administration on Aging*. Unpublished, 1978.

———. "Factors Affecting Care of the Patient: Clients, Government Policy, Role of the Family and Social Attitudes." *Journal of the American Geriatrics Society* 21:394–397, 1973.

———. "Sociological Factors of Aging Significant to the Clinician." *Journal of the American Geriatrics Society* 17:284–288, 1969.

———. *The Health of Older People: A Social Survey*. Cambridge, Mass.: Harvard University Press, 1962.

Shanas, E., and Maddox, G. L. "Aging, Health, and the Organization of Health Resources." In *Handbook of Aging and the Social Sciences*, pp. 592–618. Ed. by R. Binstock and E. Shanas. New York: Van Nostrand Reinhold, 1976.

Shuval, J. T. *Social Functions of Medical Practice*. San Francisco: Jossey-Bass, 1970.

Simon, A., and Cahan, R. "The Acute Brain Syndrome in Geriatric Patients." In *Acute Psychotic Reaction*, pp. 8–21. Ed. by W. Mendel and L. Epstein. Washington, D.C.: Psychiatric Research Report, 1963.

Sommer, R. *Personal Space*. Englewood Cliffs, N.J.: Prentice-Hall, 1969.

Sorenson, J. R. "Biomedical Innovation, Uncertainty, and Doctor-Patient Interaction." *Journal of Health and Social Behavior* 15:366–374, 1974.

Spence, D. L., Feigenbaum, E. M., Fitzgerald, F., and Roth, J. "Medical Student Attitudes Toward the Geriatric Patient." *Journal of the American Geriatrics Society* 16:976–983, 1968.

Stern, K., Smith, J., and Frank, M. "Mechanisms of Transference and Countertransference in Psychotherapeutic and Social Work with the Aged." *Journal of Gerontology* 8:328–332, 1953.

Sternback, R., and Tursky, B. "Ethnic Differences Among Housewives in Psychophysical and Skin Potential Reponses to Electric Shock." *Psychophysiology* 1:241–246, 1965.

Stevens, R. *American Medicine and the Public Interest.* New Haven: Yale University Press, 1971.

Stimson, G. V. "Interaction Between Patients and General Practitioners in the United Kingdom." In *The Doctor-Patient Relationship in the Changing Health Scene*, pp. 69–84. Ed. by E. B. Gallagher. Washington, D.C.: DHEW Pub. No. 78-183, 1978.

Suchman, E. "Stages of Illness and Medical Care." *Journal of Health and Human Behavior* 6:114–128, 1965.

Sudnow, D. *Passing On.* Englewood Cliffs, N.J.: Prentice-Hall, 1967.

Sussman, M. B.,Caplan, E. K., Haug, M. R., and Stern, M. R. *The Walking Patient.* Cleveland: The Press of Case Western Reserve University, 1967.

Szasz, T. S., and Hollender, M. H. "A Contribution to the Philosophy of Medicine: The Basic Models of the Doctor-Patient Relationship." *Archives of Internal Medicine* 94:585–592, 1956.

Thompson, P. "Understanding the Aged." *Journal of the American Geriatric Society* 13 (Oct.):893–899, 1965.

Tindale, J. A., and Marshall, V. W. "A Generational Conflict Perspective for Gerontology." In *Aging in Canada: Social Perspectives*, pp. 43–50. Ed. by V. M. Marshall. Toronto: Fitzhenry and Whiteside, 1979.

Tissue, P. "Downward Mobility in Old Age." *Social Problems* 18:67–77, 1970.

Trussell, R. E., Morehead, M. A., and Ehrlich, J. *Quantity, Quality and Costs of Medical and Hospital Care Secured by a Sample of Teamster Families in the New York Area.* New York: Columbia University School of Public Health and Administrative Medicine, 1962.

Twaddle, A. C. "Health Decisions and Sick Role Variations: An Exploration." *Journal of Health and Social Behavior* 10:105–115, 1969.

U.S. Bureau of the Census. Final Report. *Census of Population: 1970 General Social and Economic Characteristics.* U.S. summary issued 1972. Washington, D.C.: Government Printing Office, PC(1)–CI, 1972.

————. Current Population Report. *1976 Survey of Institutionalized Persons: A Study of Persons Receiving Long Term Care.* Washington, D.C.: Government Printing Office, Series P–23, No. 69, 1978.

————. Current Population Report. Washington, D.C.: Government Printing Office, Series 25, No. 870, 1980.

U.S. Department of Labor. *Manpower Report.* Washington, D.C.: U.S. Government Printing Office, 1967.

U.S. General Accounting Office. Comptroller General's Report to the Congress. *The Well-Being of Older People in Cleveland, Ohio.* Washington, D.C.: United States General Accounting Office, HRD–77–70, Apr. 19, 1977.

Vachon, M. "Staff Stress in Care of the Terminally Ill." *Quality Review Bulletin* 5:5 (May):13–17, 1979.

Vachon, M., Lyall, W., and Freeman, S. "Measurement and Mangagement of Stress in Health Professionals Working with Advanced Cancer Patients." *Death Education* 1:365–375, 1978.

Veatch, R.M. "Voluntary Risks to Health." *Journal of the American Medical Association* 243:50–55, 1980.

Verwoerdt, A. *Clinical Geropsychiatry.* Baltimore: Williams and Wilkins, 1976.

von Bertalanffy, L. "Chance or Law." In *Beyond Reductionism*, pp. 56–84. Ed. by A. Koestler and J. R. Smythies. New York: Macmillan, 1969.

———. *General System Theory*. New York: Braziller, 1968.

———. *Problems of Life*. New York: John Wiley & Sons, 1952.

Waitzkin, H. B. "A Marxist View of Medical Care." *Annals of Internal Medicine* 89:264–278, 1978.

———. "Latent Functions of the Sick Role in Various Institutional Settings." *Social Science and Medicine* 5:45–71, 1971.

Waitzkin, H. B., and Stoeckle, J. D. "Information Control and Micropolitics of Health Care: Summary of an Ongoing Research Project." *Social Science and Medicine* 10:263–276, 1976.

Waitzkin, H. B., and Waterman, B. *The Exploitation of Illness in Capitalist Society*. New York: Bobbs-Merrill, 1974.

Wan, T. "Access to Care, Health Status and Health Services Utilization of Noninstitutionalized Older Persons in Low-Income Urban Areas." Mimeographed. College Park, Md.: University of Maryland, n.d.

Weiss, P. "The System of Nature and the Nature of Systems. Empirical Holism and Practical Reductionism Harmonized." In *Toward a Man-Centered Medical Science*, pp. 17–64. Ed. by K. E. Schaefer, H. Hensel, and R. Brady. Mt. Kisco: Futura, 1977.

———. "The Living System: Determinism Stratified." In *Beyond Reductionism*, pp. 3–55. Ed. by A. Koestler and J. R. Smythies. New York: Macmillan, 1969.

———. "1 + 1 = 2. When One Plus One Does Not Equal Two." In *The Neurosciences: A Study Program*, pp. 801–821. Ed. by G. Quarton, T. Melechuk, and F. O. Schmidt. New York: Rockefeller University Press, 1967.

———. "Tierisches Verhalten als 'Systemsreaktion': Die Orientiering der Ruhestellungen von Schmetterlingen (Vanessa) gegen Licht und Schwerkraft." *Biologia General* 1:168–248, 1925.[Animal Behavior as System Reaction: Orientation Toward Light and Gravity in the Resting Postures of Butterflies (Vanessa)]. In *General Systems. Yearbook of the Society for General Systems Research IV*, pp. 1–44. Ann Arbor, Mich.: Society for the Advancement of General Systems Theory, 1959.

———. "The Biological Basis of Adaptation," In *Adaptation*, pp. 1–22. Ed. by J. Romano. Ithaca, N.Y.: Cornell Press, 1949.

———. "The Problem of Cell Individuality in Development." *The American Naturalist* 74:34–46, 1940.

Wilson, C., Banks, J., Mapes, R., and Korte, S. "Assessment of Prescribing: A Study in Operational Research." In *Problems and Progress in Medical Care*, pp. 173–201. Ed. by G. McLachlan. Oxford, England: Oxford University Press for the Nuffield Provisional Hospitals Trust, 1964.

Wilson, R. N. "Patient-Practitioner Relationships." In *Handbook of Medical Sociology*, pp. 273–295. Ed. by H. Freeman, S. Levine, and L. Reeder. Englewood Cliffs, N.J.: Prentice-Hall, 1963.

Wilson, R. N., and Bloom, S. "Patient-Practitioner Relationships." In *Handbook of Medical Sociology*, 2nd ed., pp. 315–339. Ed. by H. Freeman, S. Levine, and L. Reeder. Englewood Cliffs, N.J.: Prentice-Hall, 1972.

Wolfe, S. "The Social Responsibility of the Physician in Prescribing Mind-Affecting Drugs." In *Social Aspects of the Medical Use of Psychotropic Drugs*, pp. 53–62. Ed. by R. Copperstock. Toronto: Alcoholism and Drug Addiction Research Foundation of Ontario, 1974.

Wolfe, S., and Badgley, R. F. *The Family Doctor*. Toronto: Macmillan, 1973.

Woods, R., and Britton, P. "Psychological Approaches to the Treatment of the Elderly." *Age and Aging* 6 (May):104–112, 1977.

Wortman, C.B., and Dunkel-Shetter, C. "Interpersonal Relationships and Cancer: A Theoretical Analysis." *Journal of Social Issues* 35(1):120–155, 1979.

Zborowski, M. "Cultural Components in Response to Pain." *Journal of Social Issues* 8:16–30, 1952.

Zola, I. K. "In the Name of Health and Illness: On Some Socio-Political Consequences of Medical Influence." *Social Science and Medicine* 9:83–87, 1975.

———. "Culture and Symptoms—An Analysis of Patients' Presenting Complaints." *American Sociological Review* 31:615–630, 1966.

INDEX

Index

Abdellah, F. G., 155
Abramson, L. Y., 182
Activism, therapeutic, 111–114
Affective neutrality, Parsons' concept
　of, 24
Affective relationship of doctor and
　patient, 105–111, 115–116
Ageism, *xviii*
Aging process, attribution of symptoms
　to, 75–78
Alliances, *see* Coalitions
Alonzo, A. A., 32
American Medical Association, first
　code of ethics of, 28
Andersen, R., 75, 151
Anderson, F., *xviii*, 43
Anderson, O. W., 75, 151
Antonovsky, A., 33, 115, 116
Appointments, compliance and keeping
　of, 102
Arluke, A., 28
Artiss, K., 110
Auerbach, M., *xviii*
Authority relationship, 95, 97–105
　in the biomedical and psychosocial
　　spheres, 98–100, 114–116
　charismatic, 105
　compliance and, 100–105, 115
　conflict and negotiation in, 103–105
　mutual participation model of, 98
　negotiation of, 97–98, 103–105

Badgley, R. F., 101
Balint, M., 101
Baresi, C. M., 184
Baric, L., 71
Barker, R., 72

Barriers to doctor-patient relationship,
　35–52
　communication gap as, 49
　environmental, 46
　financing as, 49–50
　gerontologist's view of, 37–41
　patient-generated, 39–40, 45–46
　patient's view of, 47–52
　physician-generated, 40–45
　physician's view of, 42–46
　quality of care and, 48–49
Bauman, B. O., 27
Becker, H. S., 96
Beeson Committee, 174–175
Benedict, R., 166
Bengston, V. L., 192
Ben-Sira, Z., 98, 177*n*
Bercanovic, E., 27
Bias, R. R., 68
Bice, T. W., 106
Biomedical model, 3–5, 9–10, 14–15, 32
　authority relationship and, 98–99
　compliance and, 100–101
Biopsychosocial model, 3–21, 44
Bloom, S.W., 25, 96, 98, 118*n*, 149, 160,
　170*n*, 181, 183
Bloor, M. J., 96, 118*n*
Bogdonoff, M. D., *xix*, 69
Boreham, P., 29
Boureston, N. C., 156
Brehm, H. P., 114, 155
Breslau, L., 180, 184
Breytspraak, L. M., 111, 114, 117*n*
Brickner, P., *xviii*
Britton, P., *xviii*
Brody, E., 186
Brook, R. H., 150